Delivery and Deficiency:

Health and Health care in Tibet

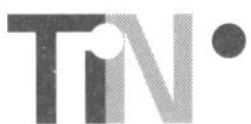

Tibet Information Network

London 2002

Printed in England
Published by Tibet Information Network (TIN), November 2002

Design & Typesetting
Jane Bartlett & Matthew Ward

ISBN: 0-9541961-3-9

Delivery and Deficiency:
Health and Health care in Tibet

Tibet Information Network (TIN):

UK HEAD OFFICE:

City Cloisters,
188-196 Old Street
London EC1V 9FR UK

tel: +44 (0)20 7814 9011
fax: +44 (0)20 7814 9015

US OFFICE:

TIN USA
PO Box 2270
Jackson WY83001

tel: +1 307 733 4670
fax: +1 307 739 2501

tin@tibetinfo.net — www.tibetinfo.net — tinusa@wyoming.com

TIN• Tibet Information Network...

culture
economy
education
environment
health
leaders
media
policies
prisoners
propaganda
religion
tourism
women

Tibet Information Network (TIN) is an independent news service and research organisation that gathers and disseminates information about the situation in Tibet. Based in London with field teams in India and Nepal, TIN monitors political, social, economic, environmental, and human rights conditions in Tibet, and then publishes this information in the form of regular news updates (via email and the web), special reports, briefing papers and specialist publications. TIN's information comes from a variety of sources both inside and outside Tibet, official and informal, as well as from its own fieldwork with Tibetan refugees, and from the monitoring of established Chinese, Tibetan and international media.

TIN's primary objective is to provide a systematic, comprehensive and impartial news, research and information service, for development agencies, governments, and non-governmental and international organisations, as well as journalists, academics, human rights groups and other interested parties. Over the last 15 years TIN has gained a worldwide reputation for reliable fact-based reporting and expert analysis of conditions and developments in present-day Tibet.

In 1996 – nine years after it was first established – TIN was registered as a charity in the UK under the title "Tibet Information Network Trust", with the following stated aims:

- *to advance the education of the public about Tibet and its people by undertaking, promoting and commissioning research into conditions and developments in and relating to Tibet*
- *to disseminate the results of such research to the general public, non-governmental organisations, inter-governmental organisations, governments, parliamentarians, the media and scholars in the UK and throughout the world.*

Tibet Information Network Trust is registered as a charity (no. 1057648) in the UK, as a limited company (no. 3226281) in England and Wales, and as a 501(c)(3) tax-exempt non-profit organisation in the USA

Acknowledgements

TIN would not have been able to compile this report without the assistance and support of many people – particularly health professionals, both Western and Tibetan, who have worked in Tibet. Due to the nature of their work, many have asked not to be named. We would however like to take this opportunity to thank them for their guidance and advice, and their concern for accuracy and objectivity.

TIN would also like to thank Jane Caple, former colleague, for her insightful comments and tireless support; Gabriel Lafitte for the flow of invaluable research materials and extremely constructive criticism; and Andrew Fischer for his generous last-minute help. A big thank you also to Tibet Images and Barefoot Images, as well as the individual photographers who provided us with informative and sensitive photographs from Tibet. This includes the *'migou'* – for his images, expertise and enthusiasm.

The researching, writing and production of this report was greatly assisted by the wealth of material collected and pre-processed by TIN's field teams in Nepal and India; the dedication and many hours of proof-reading provided by colleagues in the London office (and further south-west); as well as the participation of TIN Trustees John Bray, Pierre Robert and Colina MacDougall. Jane Bartlett deserves a particular word of thanks for her invaluable inspiration, energy and unstinting hard work in the planning and production of this volume.

The production of this report – as with other TIN publications – relies upon the many anonymous individuals who provide us with information about the situation on the ground and who, despite the inherent risks and dangers, provide the first-hand accounts that offer a powerful insight into what these issues mean to ordinary Tibetans. We are unable to acknowledge these sources publicly, but would like to express our profound gratitude to them.

Similarly TIN would like to express its utmost gratitude for the financial support that has made possible much of the research included this report, this includes donations from The Staples Trust; the Swedish International Development Co-operation Agency (SIDA); the National Endowment for Democracy (NED); The Barrow Cadbury Trust; the American Himalayan Foundation; the Ruben and Elisabeth Rausing Trust; and The Department for International Development Co-operation, Finland; as well as anonymous benefactors from the UK, France, the Netherlands and USA.

Contents

Notes	(Geography, Statistics and Sources)	6	
Preface		7	
Introduction		9	
Chapter One	**The health care system in China and Tibet**		**10-27**
	Overview: The Chinese context	11	
	Law and policy on health care	14	
	Structure of health care provision in Tibet	16	
	The unreliability of data	20	
	A shortage of qualified workers	21	
	Health care in Kham	22	
	Training and salaries	24	
	Life as a rural doctor	27	
Chapter Two	**Funding and access to health care in Tibet**		**28-41**
	Drugs and injections: their cost and use	32	
	Hospital conditions and neglect of equipment	34	
	Access to affordable health care	35	
	The right to health	37	
	Health care in Lhasa	38	
	Tibetan involvement in health projects	39	
	Tradition and modernity: Tibetan traditional medicine	40	
Chapter Three	**Factors affecting health and health care in Tibet**		**42-53**
	Major health problems in Tibet	44	
	Hygiene and its link to health	47	
	Nutrition, dietary practices and sustainability	48	
	Lack of education on health and nutrition	53	
Chapter Four	**Poverty and health**		**54-65**
	The east-west divide	56	
	Poverty, health and development	57	
	Health in a macroeconomic context	60	
	The eradication of disease	61	
	Malnutrition and stunting	61	
	Tuberculosis	64	
Chapter Five	**Mother and child health**		**66-73**
	Divinations and disease	69	
	Infant and maternal mortality	69	
	Sexually transmitted infections	71	
	Reproductive health	72	
Chapter Six	**Strategies and prevention**		**74-85**
	The treatment of Iodine Deficiency Disorders	75	
	Kashin-Beck ('Big Bone') disease	79	
	The plague	80	
	HIV and AIDS	83	
Conclusion		87	

Note on geographical references

Throughout this book TIN refers to the units of political geography currently set up under Chinese administration. TIN recognises that many geographical labels in modern use do not adequately reflect traditional Tibetan views on regional nomenclature, or on political administration.

The Tibet Autonomous Region (TAR) (Chi: Xizang Zizhiqu) was set up by the Chinese government in 1965, and covers the area of Tibet west of the Yangtse River which was previously under the jurisdiction of the Dalai Lama's government, and is often referred to as 'central Tibet' in English. After 1949, other Tibetan-inhabited areas were incorporated into the neighbouring Chinese provinces of Qinghai, Gansu, Sichuan and Yunnan. Where Tibetan communities were said to have 'compact inhabitancy' in these provinces, they were designated Tibetan autonomous prefectures (TAP).

The term 'Tibet' in this report is used ethnographically, referring not only to the TAR but to the aggregate of Tibetan inhabited areas under the People's Republic of China (PRC). Tibetan names will be used to refer to administrative entities designated 'Tibetan autonomous' by China.

Note on statistics and sources

The scarcity of reliable data has to be taken into account when attempting to assess the population's state of health and health care provision in Tibet. Caution is particularly required when assessing official Chinese statistics; even senior Chinese leaders and the official press have admitted that statistics provided by central bodies are frequently unreliable. A further problem is the general shortage of available data categorised by ethnic group, which makes it difficult to assess the health status of Tibetans.

Preface

The issues of health and health care in Tibet have been a matter of great concern among Tibet observers for many years, prompting TIN to launch a series of reports on this subject – "Delivery and Deficiency" being the first volume in that series.

Western allopathic medicine arrived in Tibet in the early 20th century, with the establishment of a few, scattered health stations. These were run either by British diplomatic officers stationed in central Tibet, or Christian missionaries who had based themselves at the outer fringes of the Tibetan plateau – for example in the Chumbi Valley, just across the border to Sikkim and India, or in more significant numbers in eastern Tibet. Apart from that, the indigenous medical science (Tib: sowa rigpa) which is nowadays known as Traditional Tibetan Medicine (TTM), remained the only known type of medicine until the middle of the 20th century. Despite the fact that TTM is today regarded as a highly sophisticated medical system, at that time, although there were a fair number of trained traditional doctors (*amchis*), Tibet had no organised and universally accessible health care system, in the modern sense.

Directly after the incorporation of Tibet into the People's Republic of China (PRC) in the early 1950s, the first systematic drive to institute a modern health care infrastructure was launched, with the building of a few hospitals and health stations for the practising of allopathic medicine. Whereas in China spectacular progress has been made in the area of public health – for instance the eradication of diseases that were historically endemic to the country, through wide-scale vaccination campaigns – the achievements in Tibet appear, even today half a century later, to be unsatisfactory, a point which even the Chinese authorities acknowledge. Recent policies that have resulted in the privatisation of the medical sector have caused considerable problems across the PRC, and have had particularly disastrous consequences in the poor western regions including Tibet, creating a situation partially similar to the poorest developing countries.

This first volume explores the complex issue of health and health care in Tibet in the broadest sense, pointing to specific problems and diseases, and the general challenges of establishing a modern health care system in Tibet, as well as analysing general policies and their impact at the grass-roots level. It sets the foundation for further reports on issues including the involvement of Western NGOs in the health care system, the practice and use of Tibetan medicine (TTM), and the epidemiology of HIV/AIDS.

Thierry Dodin, Director of TIN

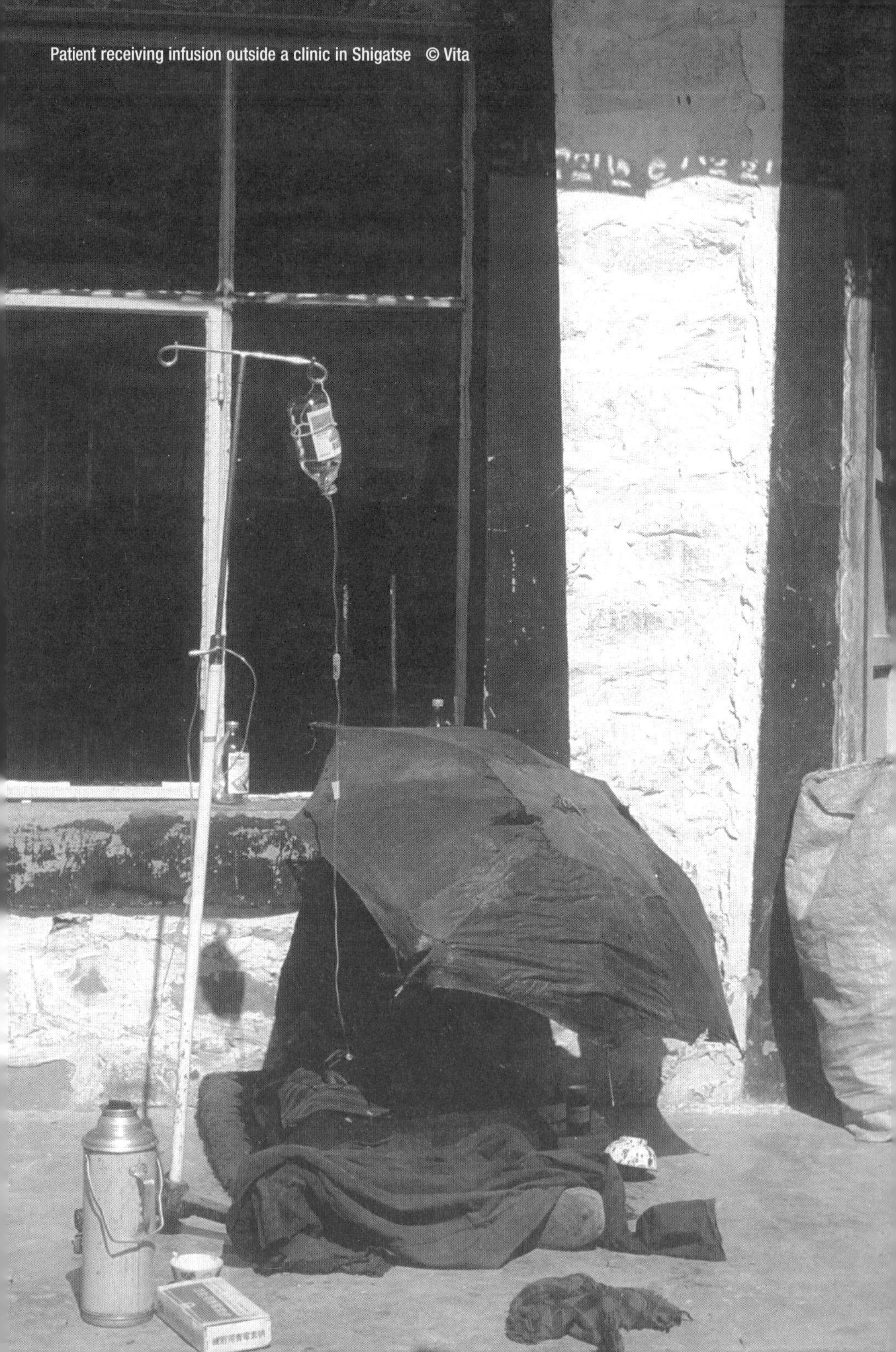

Patient receiving infusion outside a clinic in Shigatse © Vita

Introduction

Health and health care in Tibet are among the worst in the vast territory controlled by the People's Republic of China (PRC). There is a high incidence of diseases resulting from malnutrition (stunted growth, and skin and bone disorders including rickets. There have been occasional outbreaks of plague, and many people suffer from Iodine Deficiency Disorders (IDD) leading to retardation and goitres. Inadequate health care at the grass-roots level is a causal factor in rates of child and infant mortality – and deaths during child-birth – that are so high that in this regard Tibet can be categorised as one of the least developed regions on earth. The Tibet Autonomous Region (TAR) has the highest rate of tuberculosis in the PRC, and one of the highest incidences in the world of the rare Kashin-Beck (Big Bone) disease, which causes birth deformities and stunted growth. Likewise, the numbers of people suffering from blindness is higher than in most regions of the world.

This report aims to provide an overview of the health and health care situation in Tibet today based on scientific data, NGO reports and first-hand testimonies. The first two chapters establish the political and socio-economic context of the general health system in the PRC, and examine the implementation of health care policy, describing problems and challenges faced by health care workers in the field. Evidence from Tibet indicates that spending on technology, such as X-ray machines, is often prioritised over spending on basic facilities, such as running water and electricity. There is a severe shortage of village and township level health workers, and their training is neglected by the authorities. The report also analyses the key issue of access to health care for Tibetans. The failure of the health system to reach remote rural areas, coupled with prohibitive medical costs, is, for example, resulting in large numbers of Tibetan children dying from illnesses and easily treatable conditions such as diarrhoea, dysentery and pneumonia. The report also describes the major factors contributing to ill-health in Tibet, such as poor hygiene and sanitation, and inadequate nutrition. It explores the link between poverty and ill-health by summarising how poverty, particularly in rural areas, can be both a cause and consequence of poor health. Poor people are much more susceptible to disease because of lack of access to clean water and sanitation, good housing, medical care, information about preventive health care and adequate nutrition. Fees for the treatment of serious disease or illness can push Tibetans, particularly those from rural communities, deeper into a 'poverty trap' from which it is difficult to recover, forcing them into debt or the sale or mortgaging of assets such as their land and livestock.

The final two chapters focus on mother and child health, including reproductive health, and assess statistics on infant and child mortality in Tibet. This part of the report also highlights some of the most serious conditions found in Tibet – Kashin-Beck (Big Bone) Disease, IDDs, the plague and the growing threat of an HIV/AIDS epidemic – and includes comment on how delays in the implementation of preventive strategies could prove extremely damaging in the long-term.

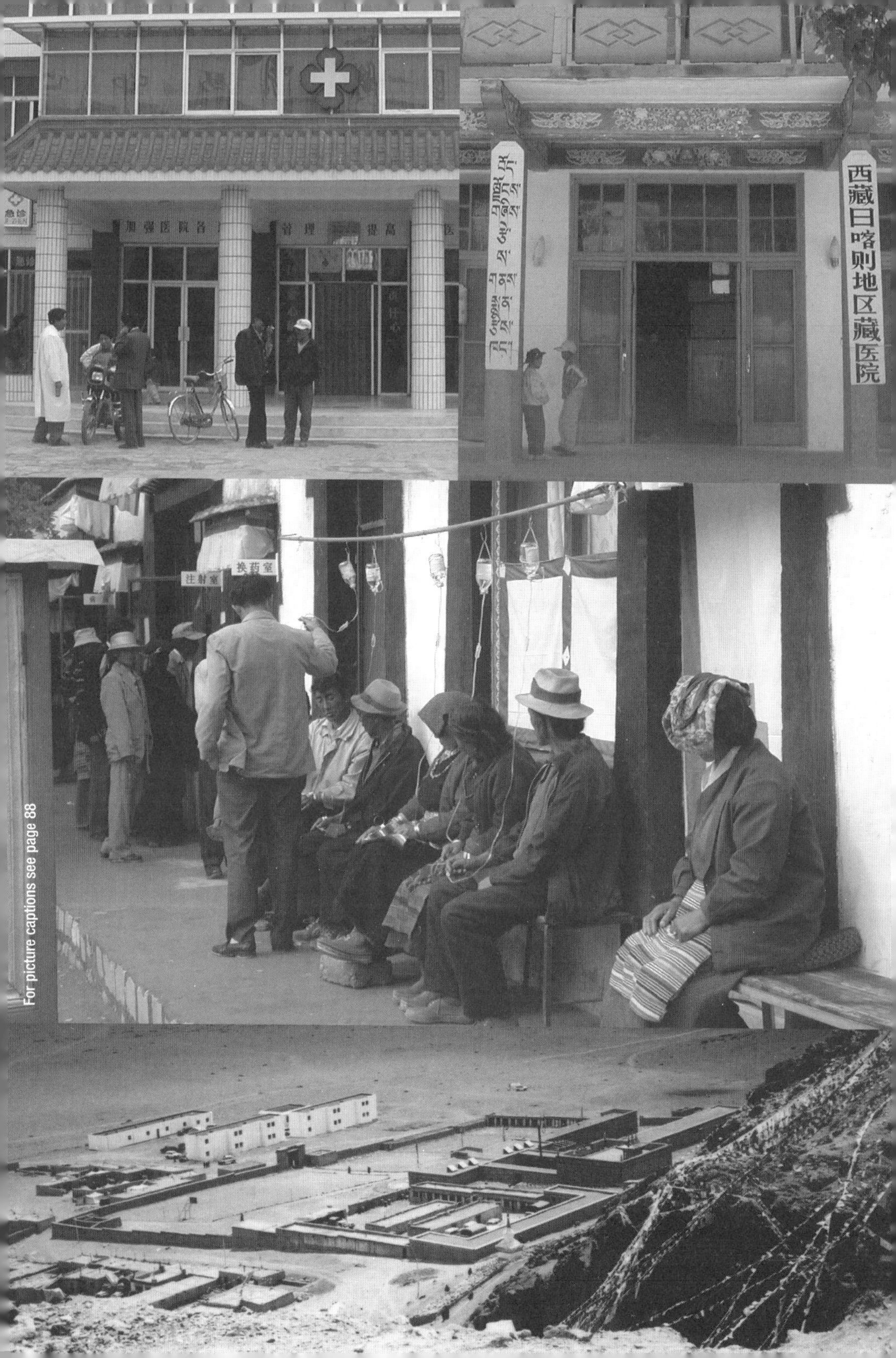

For picture captions see page 88

Chapter One

The health care system in China and Tibet

"It is an odd complaint to make of a Communist state but health and education are the two areas where most Chinese experience a lack of state intervention and a need for public services."

– Jasper Becker, China correspondent and author[1]

"The system [in Tibet] came as a surprise to me – I expected that health and education would be high priorities for a Communist government. But my experience in Tibet indicated the opposite, that they are not high priorities – sometimes there are cases when unless the foreign aid organisation agrees to provide a Landcruiser or two for local officials, there's no way they're going to be able to operate in the area."

– a Western health professional who has worked in the TAR

Overview: The Chinese context

When the Chinese Communist Party (CCP) came to power in 1949, China had undergone decades of war and revolution. Poverty was widespread and the majority of the population was uneducated in standards of health and hygiene. During the Guomindang (Nationalist) regime prior to 1949, there had been a basic medical structure in place – foreign missionaries and some Western-trained Chinese doctors worked in a number of modern hospitals, particularly in urban areas. But the majority of the population of the People's Republic of China (PRC) lacked awareness of basic issues of health and sanitation, and finances and trained personnel were in short supply. From 1949 onwards, the CCP launched a series of nationwide 'patriotic health movements' aimed at explaining the link between sanitation and health, eliminating pests, and providing immunisation which brought infections such as measles, diptheria and polio under control. During the 1960s and '70s, 'barefoot doctors', who usually had between 3 to 6 months' health training, brought minimal health care within the reach of the poorest rural communities.

1 From: "The Chinese" (John Murray 2000)

In the early years of Communist rule, the Party had valued professional expertise – such as Chinese, Western or Soviet trained doctors. But the politicisation of society resulting from a series of ideological campaigns instigated by Mao Zedong from the late 1950s onwards reversed this perception. Due to the elevation of ideology over skills, the Cultural Revolution (1966-1976) brought a loss of status for many medical and health care professionals in China and Tibet. Jasper Becker has commented that even today, both health care and education are areas where *"the intelligentsia... have yet to regain their skills and influence"* in China.[2]

From 1949 through to the 1970s, the government was responsible for social welfare in China. The introduction of the market economy and the onset of 'socialist modernisation' in the late 1970s and 1980s progressively changed this system. The burdens of financing health care shifted from the state, including state-owned enterprises, towards the provincial and local authorities through insurance schemes, and individuals. The transition was particularly severe in the rural sector as de-collectivisation cut away the financial foundation for the co-operative medical schemes.

During the 1990s, state funding of health care continued to decline in proportion to other spending, during the years of economic reform when the Party focused on fast-track economic development, and the costs of health care increased. In rural China hospital care costs up to seven times the net monthly income of a poor household.[3] According to the World Bank,[4] household surveys conducted by the Ministry of Health in 30 poor counties found the costs of rural health care to have increased twice as fast as disposable incomes during 1983-1993. From 1993 to 1998, the average cost of out-patient visits rose 232% in county hospitals and 141% in township health centres, compared with increases of 60% in the overall consumer price index and 41% in the rural consumer price index. This trend has accelerated further since then, according to the World Bank. Household surveys in rural China found that 35-40% of people who reported that they had had an illness did not seek health care, with financial difficulties cited by poor people as the main reason.[5] This trend is not unique to China: the introduction of user fees for public services and the continued increase in out-of-pocket expenses for private services is constituting a major poverty trap in other parts of the developing world.[6]

2 "The Chinese", John Murray 2000
3 Yu H, Cao S, Lucas H. "Equity in the utilisation of medical services: a survey in poor rural China". IDS Bull 1997; 28:16-23, quoted in "Equity and health sector reforms: can low income countries escape the medical poverty trap?" by Margaret Whitehead, Goran Dahigren, Timothy Evans, The Lancet, Vol 358, 8 September 2001, p 833-36
4 "China, National Development and Sub-National Finance: A Review of Provincial Expenditures", May 2002. The report includes detailed findings from investigating Hesheng and Jishishan counties in Gansu, which are close to Tibetan areas including Labrang and Rebgong in the traditional Tibetan region of Amdo
5 Fu W, "Health care for China's rural poor, international policy programme", Washington: World Bank 1999 and Hao Y, Suhua
6 Lucas H, "Equity in the utilization of medical services: a survey in poor rural China" IDS Bull 1997: 28, quoted in "Equity and health sector reforms: can low income countries escape the medical poverty trap?" by Margaret Whitehead, Goran Dahigren, Timothy Evans, The Lancet, Vol 358, 8 September 2001, p 833-36

Beijing has acknowledged that the lack of a welfare safety net in China adversely affects the provision of health care: *"An investigation carried out by the Ministry of Health indicates that some farmers who fall ill are unwilling to see a doctor or get hospitalised for fear of high costs, due to the lack of an efficient medical security system. Some farmers sink into poverty due to chronic illness... The perfection of a rural medical security system and the improvement of rural medical care is crucial to the basic interest of farmers and for the stability of society... A new, social medical care security system [has] failed to fill the vacuum created by the collapse of the old one."* (China Daily, 6 December 2001).

In March 1996, the National People's Congress (NPC) approved a scheme to further develop and improve the existing rural co-operative health system – referred to as the Co-operative Medical System (CMS). The CMS involves people paying money to the authorities to cover the cost of health care provision. Implementation of the scheme varies from county to county throughout Tibet (see Chapter Two). The NPC also stated that it would develop a medical insurance system in cities and towns, combining municipality-wide, centralised funds as well as individual accounts.[7] Graham Hutchings, China specialist and author, writes: *"[*The new urban medical insurance scheme*] required citizens to contribute towards the costs of health care once provided free by their danwei or socialist work units. Few opposed the allocation of more funds for rural health care [as] few doubted that the Mainland's ailing state industries needed to shed their welfare obligations. But at the same time, few [*people*] denied that a key element of socialism – at least as far as many urban Chinese had understood it – disappeared along with free health care."*[8]

The percentage of rural residents covered by the CMS of the Mao years dropped dramatically from around 90% to less than 10% in the 1990s.[9] The current system places an excessive burden on the state, while failing to guarantee basic medical services to the majority of Chinese and Tibetans who live in rural areas of the PRC.[10] Mao Zedong attacked the urban bias of China's health policies as far back as 1965, accusing doctors of building an elite system only in towns and cities. In nearly 40 years, the balance has not been redressed. Chinese President Jiang Zemin stated in 2002 that the emphasis of health care throughout the PRC must be in the countryside, and he has prioritised the building of a rural health insurance system[11] – an indication that the state is only now beginning to come to terms with the inadequate provision of health care following de-collectivisation.

7 See China News Analysis, No 1562, 15 June 1996 "Health and Medical Insurance"
8 "Modern China: A Companion to a Rising Power" by Graham Hutchings (Penguin, 2000), p 183
9 China News Analysis, No 1562, p 9; also see reference to a paper published in 2001 by Liu Yuanli, a Harvard School of Public Health professor and Rao Keqin, Director of the Ministry of Health's Centre for Health Statistics and Information, funded by the Asian Development Bank and China's State Development and Planning Commission, quoted in "The Sickness Trap" by Susan V Lawrence, the Far Eastern Economic Review, 13 June 2002. For further details also see "Economic Reform and Health Lessons from China", the New England Journal of Medicine, Vol 335, no 8, August 1996
10 & 11 See footnotes on next page

Law and policy on health care

The broad legal framework for health care in Tibetan areas is set by the Constitution of the PRC, which places certain obligations on the state and awards certain rights to citizens. Most importantly, Chapter 1 (General Principles), Article 21 states in part:

"*The state develops medical and health services, promotes modern medicine and traditional Chinese medicine, encourages and supports the setting up of various medical and health facilities by the rural economic collectives, state enterprises and institutions and neighbourhood organisations, and promotes health and sanitation activities of a mass character, all for the protection of the people's health.*"

"*The right to material assistance from the state and society*" is given by Article 45 of the Constitution to citizens who are old, ill or disabled. The Article states that the state is to develop the necessary social insurance, relief and medical and health services.

Article 107 of the Constitution of the PRC requires local governments at and above county level to conduct administrative work concerning public health. Article 111 requires residents' or village committees to establish sub-committees for public health "*in order to manage public affairs and social services in their areas*".

The PRC Law on Regional National Autonomy (1984, amended February 2001), which applies to all regions, prefectures and counties of the PRC known as 'nationality autonomous', states that organs of self-government of national autonomous areas "*shall make independent decisions*" on developing local medical and health services and on advancing modern and traditional medicine (Article 40), and that they shall "*strive to develop exchanges and co-operation with other areas*" in public health work (and may also do so with foreign countries) (Article 42). State organs and "*economically developed areas*" are encouraged to engage in co-operation and counterpart assistance by Articles 55 and 64.

These legal obligations are expanded upon by extensive government policies that can be dealt with only briefly here. In short, since the 1994 Third Forum for Work on Tibet, all policies for Tibet have been determined within the context of twin imperatives: acceleration of development (economic and social) and suppression of political protest and pro-independence activity. The majority of investment within the parameters of the drive to develop the western regions has been in 'hard' infrastructure – railways, roads, dams, power stations and mines for resource extraction – rather than the 'soft' infrastructure of health, education and human capacity building.

10 (see previous page) See "health and medical insurance", China News Analysis, No 1562, 15 June 1996

11 (see previous page) According to a report by Susan V Lawrence in the Far Eastern Economic Revew ("The Sickness Trap", 13 June 2002) the Chinese President apparently instructed China's Minister of Health, Zhang Wenkang, to make the building of a rural health insurance system one of the Ministry's top three priorities

Current health care priorities are briefly summarised in the 10th TAR Five-Year Plan (2001-2005). This Plan states that public health in agricultural and pastoral areas, preventive health care, and development of Tibetan medicine are to be regarded as 'the centrepiece' of public health work in Tibet (this is consistent with the TAR 9th Five-Year Plan/Long-term Targets for 2010). The goals set out in the 10th Five-Year Plan include the setting up of medical and public health networks at the county and township level, and forging a system that *"combines preventive medicine with health insurance..."* While the 9th Five-Year Plan set out a target of 'basically' making primary health care available to people in rural/pastoral areas by the year 2000, with universal access being achieved by the year 2010, the 10th Five-Year Plan refers to the need to *"improve the basic health care system in agriculture and pastoral areas, and develop co-operative medicine steadily in order to get closer to solving the basic health care problem for peasants and herders"*. Overall, the language used in the 10th Five-Year Plan is remarkably vague, and there is a notable absence of specific targets, in contrast to its predecessor. Moreover, funding remains a central question. Both the 9th and 10th Five-Year Plans refer to the need to increase health care funding, without stating how or by how much.

The 'Aid Tibet' policy provides an important additional source of funds from within the PRC. Introduced in 1994 by the 3rd Forum for Work on Tibet as part of efforts to accelerate development in the TAR, the 'Aid Tibet' policy is designed to encourage and facilitate investment and aid for specific projects (including public health projects) by central departments and individual provinces and municipalities, with a view to strengthening national cohesion of the health system. A system for the initiation and management of health care projects at regional and prefectural level was outlined in the 1995 "Health Aid to Tibet Management Regulations".[12] Regulation 2 sets out the aim of health aid to Tibet as *"raise the overall capacity of Tibet's medical treatment, prevention, healthcare, education and research by means of support from the health systems in the interior and the efforts of Tibet's front-line health staff and workers".* The 3rd National Health Aid to Tibet Work Forum was held in May 2002. In his speech to the Forum, the Minister of Health summarised the work carried out since 1994, and remarked that not only had Aid Tibet catered for Tibet's special difficulties but that it had also safeguarded 'unity of the nationalities', and 'unity and stability of the Motherland'. In another speech at the Forum, the Deputy Minister of Health reportedly referred to a need for a higher level of targeting *[zhenduixing]* for projects and to the need to listen to local cadres and make plans according to the real situation.[13]

12 Passed 9 October 1995; http://jkcj.51.net/zcfg/wsfg/yz/031.htm

13 *"Yao zai chongfen tingqu dangdi ganbu qunzhong yijian de jichu shang, tichu fuhe dangdi shiji de duikou zhihuan jihua... yao jinxing kexue, renzhen de kexinxing lunzheng, quebao xiangmu jiancheng hou fahui yingyou de xiaoyi"*, report on points made by deputy minister of health Wang Longde at the 3rd National Forum on Health Aid to Tibet, www.moh.gov.cn

Many of Tibet's problems are similar to those in other poor rural areas of China, for example, the shortage of appropriately skilled personnel, particularly at township and village level. The (national) Development Outline for Health Personnel 2001-2015[14] distinguishes between the west, central and eastern regions of China in the targets it sets, and includes specific plans to 'develop' skilled health personnel in the western regions.[15] Approximately 600 county and township health management cadres are to be trained for the western regions during the 10th National Five-Year Plan period (2001-2005), and by 2015, all village doctors in rural areas of the western regions are to have surpassed the technical middle school level of education. Attempts are also to be made to 'urge and entice' town health personnel to go and work for community health organisations, and to organise about 300 outstanding medical graduates to participate in 'development of the west'.[16] Indeed, one of the priorities of the national campaign to develop China's western regions has been to respond to the regional shortage of skilled technical personnel by encouraging migration of such personnel from eastern China, and in the longer term also to provide training and development of local personnel. These stated aims frequently serve to legitimise the influx of Chinese migrants into Tibetan areas. Thus, overall national policy – and specific policy relating to the western regions of China – is highly relevant to the examination of health policy in Tibet.

Structure of health care provision in Tibet

> *"The best way forward [in developing an effective health care service] is on two tracks. One is investing in the health system – to make it strong enough, and well-funded enough, and with the right priorities to deliver a relatively small number of essential interventions. The other is by complementary steps in education and in broader institutional advances, such as community involvement, so that the poor can effectively get access to and are motivated to seek out these essential interventions."*
>
> – The Commission on Macroeconomics and Health,
> report to the World Health Organisation (WHO), December 2001

The availability of medical treatment and the standard of hospitals and clinics varies widely not only from prefecture to prefecture but also within counties and townships in all Tibetan areas. The system generally operates on several levels – prefecture, county, township and village. In the first tier of the system, village health workers

14 *Zhongguo 2001-2015 nian weisheng renli fazhan gangyao,* 2002-35, Ministry of Health, 27 April 2002, www.moh.gov.cn
15 Development Outline, section 4(7), Policy Measures: *"Greatly strengthen development of skilled personnel in the western regions, carry out some practical things for development of skilled personnel in the western regions"*
16 Development Outline, section 4(7)

diagnose and treat patients, prescribe pharmaceuticals and refer patients to higher levels of services. Village health workers in some areas also take responsibility for preventive services, such as children's immunisation under the direction of the Anti-Epidemic Station, and ante-natal and post-natal care.

In a group of villages surveyed by a Western non-governmental organisation (NGO), all the village health workers had only primary level school education; the older ones were previously 'barefoot' doctors and then received rudimentary training as general practitioners at county and prefecture levels for about half a year (see "Training of Tibetan health workers" in this chapter). Their salaries are very low. In general, the utilisation of village clinics is higher than township or county hospitals due to their proximity for local communities and lower costs of medical treatment. Village health workers generally work from their homes using a medical bag that contains a standard set of basic diagnostic and injection equipment and a supply of drugs. They often visit patients in their home using a barter system to accept food as payment. Some rural health workers do not receive a salary for many months, sometimes years, due to lack of funds or mismanagement. This problem also applies to the medical profession in rural China as a whole. Many medical workers at the village level in China receive no pay, or partial pay, and must make their money from prescribing medicine. Doctors in China sometimes charge up to five times the actual cost of drugs in order to make ends meet or simply to make a profit.[17] This trend is also evident in other parts of the developing world; in a growing number of countries, profits from sales of drugs have become an important part of health-related workers' incomes, and an incentive for workers to increase sales to their maximum.[18]

The second tier of the system is the township clinic, staffed by permanent and temporary health personnel. A township is an administrative centre for a cluster of villages, based in one village and usually consisting of an administration centre, a school and a health clinic. These facilities can deliver babies, treat infections and wounds and in some areas can provide some basic examinations such as X-rays.

17 Ray Yip, UNICEF's Senior Project Officer for Health and Nutrition, said: *"This [over-charging for drugs] creates a false demand and a crisis of confidence among consumers that made them avoid treatment for fear of being duped"* (South China Morning Post, 5 July 2002). Village doctors in China and Tibet also make money from injections and intravenous drips, which they often do not know how to carry out properly. The Far Eastern Economic Review on 13 June 2002 reported that the Ningxia Health Bureau has started to take steps to keep profit-seeking doctors in check – in six counties in Ningxia that are part of a United Nations Children's Fund project, the Health Bureau has banned village doctors from giving intravenous therapy, and have also required doctors to cut back the drugs on their shelves to 80, and to forego expensive antibiotics in favour of cheaper ones. Doctors get US$7 a month each to make up for the income lost by the changes

18 See "Equity and health sector reforms: can low income countries escape the medical poverty trap?" by Margaret Whitehead, Goran Dahigren, Timothy Evans, The Lancet, Vol 358, 8 September 2001, p 833-36, which quotes as an example the paper "The role of pharmaceuticals in the privatization process in Vietnam", Soc Sci Med 1995; 41: 1325-32. The article in The Lancet reports that people in parts of rural China spend between two and five times the average daily per capita income on a typical prescription

Fees charged to patients differ widely from area to area, and so does the level of expertise available at the clinic.[19] Often, spending on equipment is prioritised over spending on basic facilities. One township clinic in Shigatse prefecture apparently has an X-ray machine, for instance, but no running water and no electricity.[20]

According to the TAR authorities, the township clinics have different functions distinguishing them from the larger county hospitals.[21] These include the following: prevention and care including immunisation and maternal and child health care, provision of curative services such as common disease treatment and family planning services with the addition of technical supervision, and rural health management, such as assisting the local government in managing the Co-operative Medical Services (CMS) programme, health monitoring, and data collection. Medicines are normally allocated to the township clinics by the county health bureau, and village doctors will approach the township clinics for medicine. Reports received by TIN indicate that the actual provision of health care in these township-level clinics is often very different to the roles they are assigned by the authorities, and in many of them, doctors are practising with very basic, often old and broken equipment and a lack of essential drugs.

The third referral level in the health care system in Tibet is generally the county, city or prefectural hospital. County hospitals are often the last points of referral for in-patient treatment of rural residents since few farmers, nomads, herders or unemployed Tibetans can afford to be treated at specialist hospitals in the cities. County hospitals in the Tibet Autonomous Region (TAR) typically have five departments – obstetrics and gynaecology, paediatrics, general surgery, internal medicine and laboratories/X-ray, as well as emergency room facilities.[22]

19 Clinics generally consist of just one room, with an adjoining room where the doctor lives and cooks their food. Some clinics have a separate room for mothers to deliver babies, and another for patients to stay overnight

20 The same phenomenon occurs throughout China. Jasper Becker notes in his book "The Chinese" (John Murray 2000) that 80% of health spending in China goes on big city hospitals that have spent money on acquiring modern equipment. By 1986, according to Becker, China had 170 computerized tomographic (CT) scanners (tomography is a method of body imaging in which the X-ray source and/or detection device rotate around the patient) and Beijing alone had bought 34, despite a shortage of qualified technicians to operate them. Seven years later, the country as a whole had 1,300 CT scanners and 200 magnetic resonance imaging machines, and hospitals in Beijing alone had more of these machines than the whole of Britain

21 There are now some counties where one township clinic has been chosen to be expanded and used as the primary referral centre before the county hospital is used. These township clinics sometimes have X-ray facilities and basic laboratory equipment

22 A European Union study summarised the structure of the TAR health-care system as follows: *"The health system in Tibet is organised in a hierarchical way with a health facility near the population functioning as the first line; the health post with the village doctor. He provides curative as well as preventive services. At the shang (Chi: xiang, or township) level, in some areas a shang doctor can be found. Here beds are available and patients can be kept under observation. At the county level a county level hospital can be found with personnel of an increased level of competence. The county hospital should provide specialised care (paediatrics, surgery, etc) and investigations should possibly be performed (X-ray, laboratory). Next to this a network of Tibetan medicine exists, with a referral hospital in Lhasa."* Commission of the European Communities" China – Feasibility Study for an Integrated Rural Development Project in Pa Nam County, Tibet", September 1994, Main Report, 20-21, quoted in ICJ report December 1997

In recent years many existing county hospitals have been expanded and new ones built, in both Tibet and China. However a health professional who has travelled widely throughout Tibetan areas told TIN that this does not appear to have led to a substantial improvement in health care provision in the region. The health worker told TIN: *"I visited one gleaming new hospital in a county town in the TAR, but all the patients were staying in an old row of dark rooms at the side of the new compound – they said it was cheaper and they could not afford the rooms in the new building. There were as usual many doctors in the new hospital but no increase in the number of patients since the hospital had opened. The situation was similar in a hospital I visited in Kardze* [Chi: Ganzi] *Tibetan Autonomous Prefecture (TAP) in Sichuan province where the only in-patient for the newly refurbished county hospital was sleeping outside in a tent because she could not afford the cost of a room in the new hospital."* In many of the county hospitals, surgery cannot be carried out because of the lack of equipment or specialised personnel, such as anaesthetists or surgeons.

Other public health services operating in addition to the three-tier system include the Maternal and Child Health Programme and family planning services, and the Epidemic Prevention Service (these areas of health and health care provision are discussed more fully in Chapters Six and Five). Private clinics also operate outside the three-tier system; many of them are not registered with their county health bureau. In many rural areas Buddhist lamas or healers provide consultations to people in their own homes.

A study based on detailed fieldwork in two poor counties of China immediately adjacent to Tibetan areas produced by the World Bank in 2002[23] concludes that the quality of health services in China is highly dependent on the financial health of the local budget. The report states: *"Each level of government finances largely its own facilities. Provincial governments support referral hospitals in the provincial capital and the institutions that supervise preventive programmes. The same applies to prefecture, county and township governments. Consequently, township health centres receive most of their very low levels of financial support from township governments. Very few resources are transferred from higher levels of government to facilities at the lower levels to support recurrent costs, although there are some earmarked grants for specific objectives and activities[...] The level of subsidy diminishes down the administrative hierarchy[...] in some of the poorer townships in Hezheng county, there were reportedly no budgetary inputs to the health sector at all."*

23 "China, National Development and Sub-National Finance: A Review of Provincial Expenditures", May 2002 which includes detailed findings from investigations in Hezheng and Jishishan counties in Gansu which are close to major Tibetan centres such as Labrang and Rebgong

The unreliability of data

> *"People in Tibet are literally frightened of speaking out. Local cadres, for instance, might be unwilling to report on a particularly bleak situation by saying that help is needed from outside – the basic line is that everything is under control. This does not create a good environment to achieve change and progress within the health system."*
>
> – Western health professional with experience in Tibet[24]

The discrepancies and unreliability of statistics in Tibet and China result, in part at least, from an unwillingness and fear, at local level, of being held accountable for poor conditions of health, such as malnutrition and high infant mortality. A Chinese official working in Tibetan areas told one Western NGO that they had been told by other officials to report that malnutrition in one area was due to *"Tibetan backwardness and lack of education"*, and not to poverty and/or failings of the health system. Another Western charity referred to a system of under-reporting of illness at various township clinics in the TAR: *"Reporting of births, well-child attendances, antenatal checks and deaths seemed relatively comprehensive at both clinic and central levels. However the official reporting system for morbidity,[25] recording anaemia, diarrhoea, pneumonia and bone/joint disorders, showed such a degree of under-reporting as to render the information meaningless."*

An experienced health professional who is familiar with the situation in Tibet told TIN that medical statistics were often produced for a particular purpose – for instance to show that Tibet needs subsidies from Beijing. The health professional told TIN of one instance: *"One advisor to the Chinese government was using invented figures to show to people from Chinese ministries how statistics could be presented, in order to seek funding from outside organisations. Later the report came back from Beijing – including exactly the same figures he'd invented. There are figures [at county level] on health but you can't see them until after they have been doctored in Lhasa."*

A former cadre from Sichuan province told TIN that when Tibetan officials are honest about the poor social conditions in their area, sometimes improvements can be made, even though the individual may face punitive measures. The Tibetan source told TIN that one Party official in a nearby township made records of the real income of local people. Because these statistics did not reflect the goals set in the plans, the official lost his position in the area. The Tibetan said: *"Even though he incurred many losses, he managed to benefit the people, because now the prefecture recognises his township as a poor area."*

24 In conversation with TIN, October 2002
25 Morbidity is a diseased condition or state; it also refers to the incidence or prevalence of a disease or of all diseases in a population

A shortage of qualified workers

The shortage of skilled medical and technical personnel in Tibet is acknowledged in the TAR 10th Five-Year Plan. In May 2002, the Deputy Minister of Health remarked at the 3rd National Forum on Health Aid to Tibet to Tibet (May 2002) that the lack of high quality health management and other skilled personnel was a 'bottle-neck' constricting development of health care in Tibet. In rural Tibet, there is a serious shortage of adequately trained village and township-level health personnel, and many skilled medical workers have left rural areas to find more lucrative work in cities.[26] A study by a Western NGO in the Shigatse (Chi: Rigaze) area of the TAR in 1998 found that there were no clinics in 165 villages surveyed, but that there were 67 village doctors working from home to cover this area, with each village health worker covering two or three villages. The NGO concluded that this lack of a clinic and facilities for the village health worker to store medicines and equipment compromised the ability of the doctor to maintain safe injection practices and to perform minor procedures in a safe, clean manner. Another NGO concluded after a similar study in the TAR that there are *"not enough personnel trained to a high level; most personnel have had mid or low-level training lasting typically 3 years or 1-6 months respectively."*[27] The Red Cross Society of China was reported by the International Commission of Jurists as stating that the areas under study *"were in desperate need of health care, where a common illness rapidly develops in chronic complication leading to life dangers"*.[28] A 1994 European Union (EU) report on health care in Tibet noted the shortage of nurses, the heavy workload of village health care workers and a lack of female doctors.[29]

The same EU report concluded that the hierarchical system was 'top-heavy' with *"relatively more doctors in the county hospital... perhaps too many... while the first-line is rather under-staffed"*. While there is clearly a problem with a lack of adequately trained medical personnel in rural Tibetan areas, over-staffing elsewhere in the health service, particularly in hospitals at the prefecture and county level, contributes to the overall inefficiency of the health service in both Tibet and China. China has made public commitments to reduce numbers of civil service personnel, including those in the health service, but there is evidence that this commitment is not being carried through in Tibetan areas or elsewhere in the PRC. Salaries account for an extremely high proportion of health spending overall, contributing to the dysfunctional nature of the health system throughout China.[30]

26 Health workers in Tibet are generally known as *amchi*. The term traditionally referred to someone who has received comprehensive medical training, but it is often now used to describe someone who has only had about 6 weeks training
27 Quoted in "Tibet: Human Rights and the Rule of Law", International Commission of Jurists, December 1997, p 230
28 Ibid, note 138, p 225
29 European Communities, Feasibility Study, Main Report 21, September 1994, quoted in ICJ report December 1997
30 See footnote on next page

Health care in Kham

In August 2001 a team led by Dr. Bruce Beattie of the charity International SOS in partnership with the charity Kham Aid surveyed clinics and hospitals along the north Sichuan-Tibet highway, in the course of a bike ride. A full report of their visits to clinics along the route, in Kardze TAP (Chi: Ganzi), Sichuan province, can be viewed at the Kham Aid website at: http://www.khamaid.org/.

An extract from the report is below:

> *"Nearly all the doctors we met or heard about during the survey were graduates of the vocational school for medicine in Guza (a small town at the eastern edge of the prefecture). The Guza school has 3 and 4-year programs, which is sufficient training to receive credentials and be assigned a job. People entering this institution are graduates only of junior middle school, which means that they have only 9 years of prior formal education and are as young as 16 or 17 [years]. Scanty training is one of the biggest problems afflicting medical care in Ganzi, but it is not unique to Ganzi or to Tibetan areas – it is common throughout rural China.*
>
> *Most of the hospitals and clinics we visited had a large staff – too large for the number of patients. This has several bad effects: first, that wages must be kept low (US$110/month for a typical doctor [sic]) to accommodate the large payroll; and second, that staff seems to take the situation as a license to be absent for long periods. In only one clinic did we actually meet the director. In the other places, the director was not around. Absence of the leader takes an obvious toll on care quality, organisation efficiency, and especially morale.*
>
> *In the past few years, across China, the government has been trying to trim the bloated civil service. A couple of years ago they were talking about eliminating one third of jobs. Yet this has proven politically difficult, and so far has not been achieved.*

30 (see previous page) A report published in May 2002 by the World Bank made various suggestions for the re-structuring of the health system in China, suggesting that Beijing should *"fundamentally reformulate health finance and clarify the public role in the health sector"* and should reassess issues of over-staffing. The World Bank recommended that Beijing should "take on a direct role in financing health care expenditures for poor households as well as poor localities... regulate user charges including imposing limits on prescription drug profits to health centres so as to minimise the incentive to over-prescribe medicines... introduce safety net provisions to ensure health coverage for poor households... address issues of overstaffing and unqualified personnel in health facilities". World Bank report, China: National Development and Sub-National Finance: A Review of Provincial Expenditures", May 2002

Except for the Dawu county hospital, hygiene at the clinics and hospitals we visited was poor. Rooms were dark and unheated, floors made of unsealed concrete, furniture battered and chipped, sheets washed and reused until they were only blood-stained rags. Ward beds had little padding. Staff housing is cramped and squalid. There was often no running water, either hot or cold. Medical practice in Ganzi relies heavily on injections and intravenous (IV) drips – this treatment being preferred by many patients. I have seen people receiving IV drips at home and spotted them walking around on the street, a friend holding the bottle overhead. Antibiotics are, by Western standards, vastly over-prescribed, being thought to cure even the common cold or flu. This mistaken view is probably common throughout China. I have seen friends who, when ill, went down to the clinic, got a shot, and then clearly expected that they would now improve – which they did, so the attitude dies hard. In every clinic, we saw a large supply of injectable drugs. At least they do use disposable needles much of the time.

Rural doctors spend a great deal of time outside their clinics making house calls. Sometimes this involves travel of a day or more. At the better clinics, women will come in to give birth, but at less hygienic ones there is no advantage in this and a doctor will probably be summoned to supervise a home birth. Typically, a woman will go in for an ultra-sound examination just once during her pregnancy.[31] *Many births take place without a doctor present, especially in remote areas.*

One of our surprising findings was the government support given to traditional medicine systems. Many Tibetans – especially older, more conservative people – prefer traditional Tibetan medicines. One reason is that they are quite a bit cheaper. By contrast, I have also met Tibetans in rural Ganzi who, when a family member is seriously ill, have bankrupted themselves to send the patient to the finest western hospitals in Chengdu. Thus there is a wide range of preference in medical care. As medical costs are prohibitive, poor families are discouraged from seeking care until the situation becomes desperate. Like elsewhere in China, Ganzi's health care system is far less accessible to ordinary people than it was 10 or 20 years ago."

31 This is not necessarily too unusual; in various Western countries such as the Netherlands many women are not offered ultra-sound during their pregnancy (although this does not mean it is not available in the West)

Training and salaries

The experience and expertise of health workers in Tibetan areas varies considerably. A survey of some of the health workers in six different counties in Shigatse prefecture in the TAR, by one Western NGO, showed that their medical experience and training ranged from several weeks or months to several years. One of the most well educated health workers in the area has 4 years of training in China, and several years working as a doctor in the prefecture. Other rural health workers in the area have no formal health training and only middle school education.

Overall the knowledge and technical competence of health workers at all levels of the system is poor, particularly at the village, township and county level. The performance of health workers reflects their lack of training, lack of follow up to any training they receive and lack of supervision. Training that does take place uses out-dated textbooks and training methods that do not provide health workers with the knowledge and/or skills to diagnose and treat diseases correctly. Township and village doctors throughout Tibet who have been interviewed by Western NGOs request additional training and/or specialist training to enable them to work more effectively.

A supervisory system is in place in many counties and is the responsibility of the county hospital and county level Public Health Bureau – which are expected to form a supervisory committee that arranges regular visits to the township clinics. However, most counties do not have a separate budget for this activity, and due to the lack of a budget for travel and field allowances for the supervisors, many township doctors report rarely if ever seeing a supervisor. Those who do see a supervisor report that rather than helping to update the health worker's technical skills they spend time explaining administrative issues relating to prescription charges and how to calculate reimbursement through the CMS system.

Salaries of health workers in central Tibetan areas can range from approximately 90 yuan (US$10.84) per month to 1200 yuan (US$144) per month, largely depending on whether they are categorised as a 'temporary' or 'permanent' health worker. Permanent workers are government employees who receive a salary, health insurance, pension and job security; they are generally health school graduates. The majority of health workers at township level and all those at village level are known as 'temporary' rather than 'permanent'. However, many of these so-called 'temporary' health workers have many years of experience in their local clinics, although they may not have formal qualifications. They earn far less than their permanent health worker colleagues.

The nationwide institutional reform of the health care system being implemented from the Ministry of Health in Beijing includes the replacement of all temporary health workers at township and county level with college graduates who have completed 3 or 4 years of health school training (this does not apply to village health workers). The director of a prefectural-level hospital in the TAR said: *"This will be a slow process and will happen over the next 5 years. Temporary workers will retire and be replaced with permanent workers. Many of the temporary workers have many years of experience although no formal health education. It would be good if there was a method of selecting those who are highly skilled and competent and re-training them to bring them up to a better educational level."*[32] Some Tibetans fear that with the replacement of temporary workers, more Chinese health workers will replace Tibetan health workers at county and township level.

In Tibet, the decision to appoint a particular health care professional is based on a several factors, not solely the person's medical expertise and credentials. Reports from Tibet indicate that just as in every other professional field in China and Tibet, good *guanxi* (connections) and political influence play an important part in gaining employment or a senior official position. One Westerner who has worked in health care in Tibet told TIN that Tibetans or Chinese are often recruited to posts in the medical profession solely because of their contacts: *"All you can say is that the [*official counterparts to Western aid organisations*] don't care about capacities, they only care about money and positions and nepotism."* Similarly, county and prefectural directors of public health services in Tibet are often rewarded with appointments simply for being a good Party member, not their medical knowledge or administrative skills.

The issue of which language is used by health professionals is crucial in both the TAR and Tibetan areas outside the TAR. Training and reference materials, and instructions on equipment and medicine, are typically in Chinese, and hence not able to be read by the majority of people at county level and below. Outside the main towns and cites most Tibetans do not understand spoken Chinese, and hence doctors need to communicate in Tibetan. A report by a Western charity operating in the TAR stated: *"Most township doctors are not bilingual, some of them can only speak Tibetan and some of them can only speak Chinese. It is difficult for them to communicate with each other and with the local people. This is especially difficult for those who only speak Chinese – even though they have a college degree, it remains difficult for them to communicate with their patients and their Tibetan colleagues. When a Chinese doctor is alone in the township clinic, local people do not go to seek her/him for help and prefer to leave or to wait for a doctor who can understand and communicate with them."*

32 Conversation with Western NGO health worker

Life as a rural doctor

The following account of the difficulties of medical practice in a nomadic area of the TAR was given to TIN by a Tibetan doctor in his thirties who left Tibet in the late 1990s:

> *"I am an ordinary pastoral doctor who studied traditional Tibetan medicine at a very early age, with experience of the practice for more than 15 years. I have neither received [equal] recognition nor medical facilities from either the county authority or from the regional administration. During my years of medical practice, I received one medical training session that was organised and funded by Western people and one training session in Lhasa that I paid for with my own money. I have not received any help or funding from the authorities.*
>
> *Regarding the so-called subsidised medical treatment in rural areas – every person is entitled to get his or her first treatment at a rate that seems to be heavily subsidised. In reality most of the medicine provided at a subsidised rate is either out-of-date or is very basic, such as pain-killers, wound solutions and water for washing wounds. This Chinese government's subsidised rate cannot satisfy the medical need of the nomads. Even pain and bleeding cannot be stopped by these subsidised medicines.*
>
> *In my region there were many people who died or who are still ill due to lack of proper medical facilities. Especially due to the snowstorms that occurred one winter, there were many people in an area I could not reach who were ill with no food; and the death rate of infants under 1 year of age increased sharply.*
>
> *[During the snowstorms] we, the private doctors, gathered to treat the people with our limited resources and medicines. Finally after many years of practice, four years ago the authority gave me only 30 yuan (US$3.61) a month to cover my medical expenses and the salary, with some out of date medicines. One of my main reasons for escaping from Tibet was that the Chinese government devalued the years of my experience and knowledge of medicines."*

A Westerner who worked in the TAR for an NGO working on health care in Tibet provided the following portrait of a typical village doctor in Tibet:[33]

> *"Mostly he is a man, he is in his late twenties and had his first training for about a month. He went to school at the age of 11 or 12 and has some difficulties in Tibetan writing. Like most of his colleagues, he had a refresher course for 2 to 3 weeks, but part of the training was in Chinese and he doesn't understand this language. He is living in a small village of about 200 people but he is responsible for other villages in the area, approximately 900 people. Everyday he is checking 15 patients, half are coming to his small house where he has no special room to do this; he also has to go to visit some of them as far away as 15-20 kilometres. For this he has to rent a horse or a bicycle or sometimes go on foot. The next regional hospital where he can refer patients to is further away and the road is especially difficult during the rainy season. So he does not have many contacts with doctors there.*
>
> *He should receive drugs every three months but they often do not arrive for 6 months. He cannot recognise labels written in Chinese or Latin and has to ask someone what it is and take notes in Tibetan. As dressing material is very expensive, he doesn't receive any. Some patients are angry with him because they think he has drugs but he doesn't want to give them out. When he has to go for immunisation, no one gives him enough syringes or vaccines, and he has to work very hard to cover his area and meet the targets for this. Apart from this immunisation work, none of his tasks are preventative.*
>
> *He is also a farmer and his medical work should not exceed 50% of his time, but often he is called out, sometimes at night, and when he goes to do immunisations, his wife needs someone to help with the farm work. He has taken some examinations and was told that he passed, but he never received the certificates, so his salary stayed at about 25 yuan (US$2.41) and is sometimes less if he doesn't complete his immunisations. He didn't choose his job but is very dedicated to the people and would like to know more in order to better serve his community."*

33 This account was written in the early 1990s but is still relevant today

For picture captions see page 88

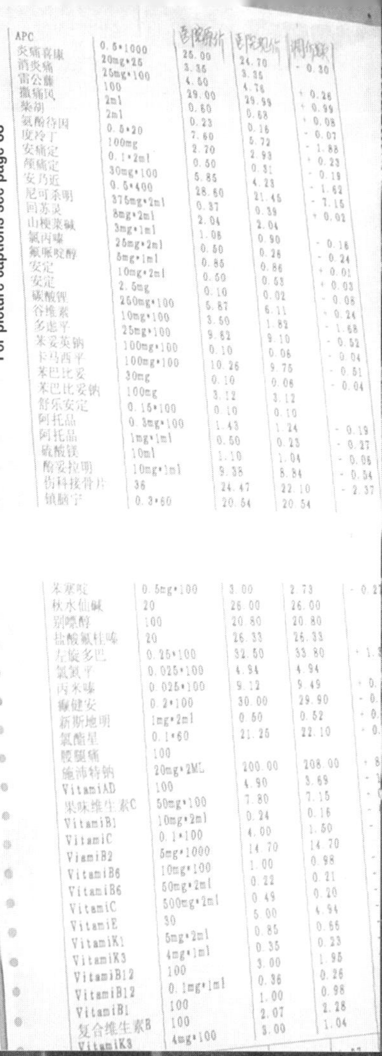

		医院原价	医院现价	调价额
APC	0.5*1000	25.00	24.70	- 0.30
炎痛喜康	20mg*25	3.35	3.35	
消炎痛	25mg*100	4.50	4.76	+ 0.26
雷公藤	100	29.00	29.99	+ 0.99
撒痛风	2ml	0.60	0.68	+ 0.08
柴胡	2ml	0.23	0.16	- 0.07
氨酚待因	0.5*20	7.60	5.72	- 1.88
度冷丁	100mg	2.70	2.93	+ 0.23
安痛定	0.1*2ml	0.50	0.31	- 0.19
颅痛定	30mg*100	5.85	4.23	- 1.62
安乃近	0.5*400	28.60	21.45	- 7.15
尼可杀明	375mg*2ml	0.37	0.39	+ 0.02
回苏灵	8mg*2ml	2.04	2.04	
山梗菜碱	3mg*1ml	1.08	0.90	- 0.16
氯丙嗪	25mg*2ml	0.50	0.26	- 0.24
氟哌啶醇	5mg*1ml	0.85	0.86	+ 0.01
安定	10mg*2ml	0.50	0.53	+ 0.03
安定	2.5mg	0.10	0.02	- 0.08
碳酸锂	250mg*100	5.87	6.11	+ 0.24
谷维素	10mg*100	3.50	1.82	- 1.68
多虑平	25mg*100	9.82	9.10	- 0.52
苯妥英钠	100mg*100	0.10	0.06	- 0.04
卡马西平	100mg*100	10.26	9.75	- 0.51
苯巴比妥	30mg	0.10	0.06	- 0.04
苯巴比妥钠	100mg	3.12	3.12	
舒乐安定	0.15*100	0.10	0.10	
阿托品	0.3mg*100	1.43	1.24	- 0.19
阿托品	1mg*1ml	0.50	0.23	- 0.27
硫酸镁	10ml	1.10	1.04	- 0.06
酚妥拉明	10mg*1ml	9.38	8.84	- 0.54
伤科接骨片	36	24.47	22.10	- 2.37
镇脑宁	0.3*60	20.54	20.54	

苯噻啶	0.5mg*100	3.00	2.73	- 0.2
秋水仙碱	20	26.00	26.00	
别嘌醇	100	20.80	20.80	
盐酸氟桂嗪	20	26.33	26.33	
左旋多巴	0.25*100	32.50	33.80	+ 1.
氯氮平	0.025*100	4.94	4.94	
丙米嗪	0.025*100	9.12	9.49	+ 0.
癫健安	0.2*100	30.00	29.90	- 0.
新斯地明	1mg*2ml	0.50	0.52	+ 0.
氯酯醒	0.1*60	21.25	22.10	+ 0.
腰腿痛	100			
施沛特钠	20mg*2ML	200.00	208.00	+ 8
VitamiAD	100	4.90	3.69	- 1
果味维生素C	50mg*100	7.80	7.15	-
VitamiB1	10mg*2ml	0.24	0.16	-
VitamiC	0.1*100	4.00	1.50	-
ViamiB2	5mg*1000	14.70	14.70	
VitamiB6	10mg*100	1.00	0.98	-
VitamiB6	50mg*2ml	0.22	0.21	-
VitamiC	500mg*2ml	0.49	0.20	-
VitamiE	30	5.00	4.94	-
VitamiK1	5mg*2ml	0.85	0.66	-
VitamiK3	4mg*1ml	0.35	0.23	-
VitamiB12	100	3.00	1.95	
VitamiB12	0.1mg*1ml	0.36	0.26	
VitamiB1	100	1.00	0.98	
复合维生素B	100	2.07	2.28	
VitamiK3	4mg*100	3.00	1.04	

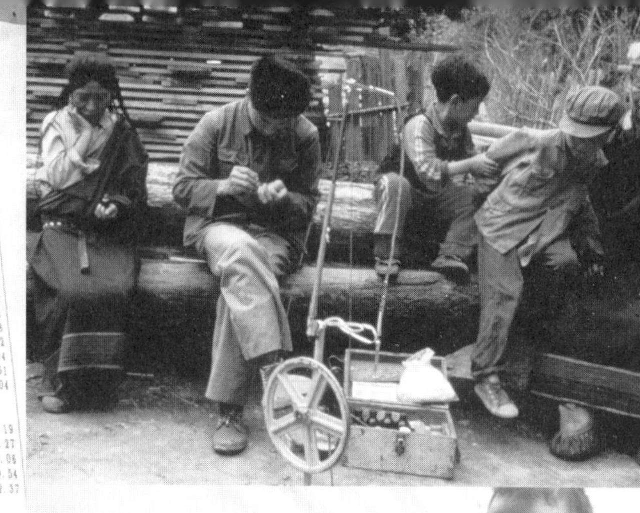

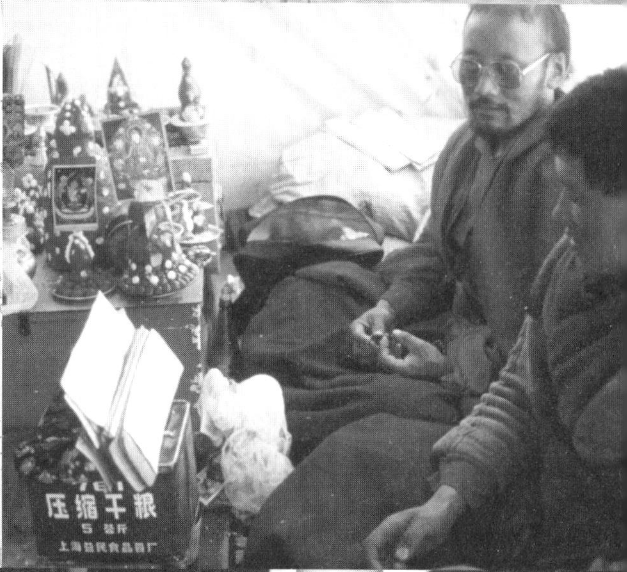

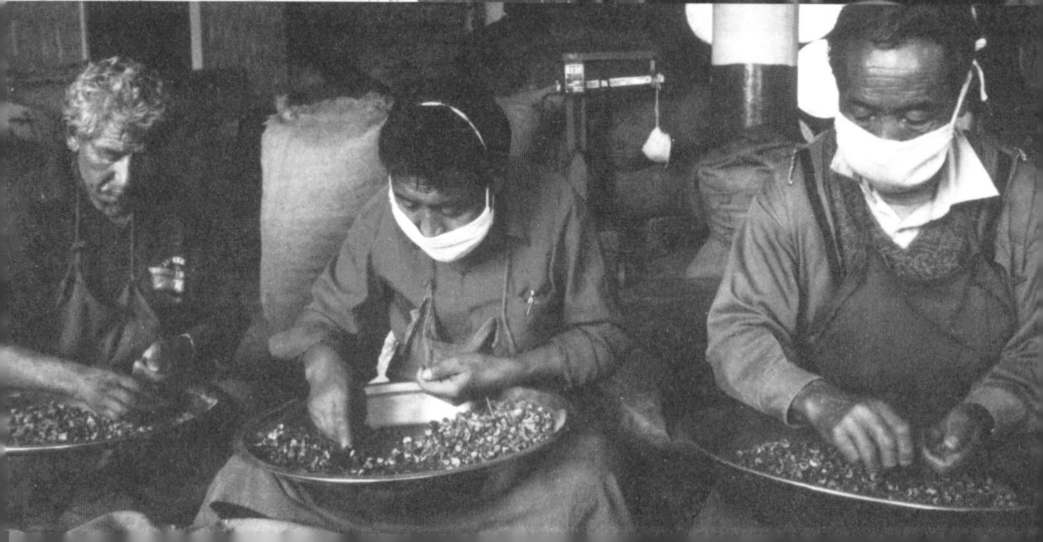

Chapter Two

Funding and access to health care in Tibet

> *"The PRC claims 'the government provides free medical care for all Tibetans.' One medical aid worker in Tibet, however, described the health care system as 'the most expensive free health care system in the world.'"*
>
> – presentation by the NGO, International League for Human Rights, to the UN Commission on Human Rights, 58th session, 2001

The 9th and 10th Five-Year Plans of the Tibet Autonomous Region (TAR) acknowledge the central question of the need to increase funding of the health system, although they do not give details of how much funding would be needed or might be available to improve health care provision in the TAR. The development of the Co-operative Medical System (CMS) in rural areas and urban medical insurance schemes, which are referred to in the TAR 10th Five-Year Plan (2001-2005), are a key element of Beijing's aims in the provision of health care throughout the People's Republic of China (PRC).[1] The ongoing development of the medical insurance system constitutes a further index of the disparities between rural and urban areas in the PRC.[2]

The nationwide reform of the health care system being implemented by Beijing involves the full implementation of the CMS, which operates on the principle of payments being made by individuals into their local health service. The individual can then use health facilities in their area and will only pay a portion of the costs for health worker visits and medication. Services that should be covered by the CMS include basic health treatment, disease prevention, maternal and child health care, health education and family planning methods. Persons not covered by the CMS system are required to pay out-of-pocket for services and medications.

1 For example, according to a Xinhuanet article on 31 December 2001, 40,000 Tibetan government cadres in the TAR had signed up for medical insurance since 1 December that year. Xinhuanet reported: *"This is expected to solve the financial difficulties for the low-income and laid-off workers when they have serious illnesses."* On 9 July 2002 the official website www.tibetinfor.com reported the setting up of *"experimental units"* of *"hospitalisation insurance system reform"* in the Lhasa area on 1 December 2001

2 Health insurance has become *"the next test of the legitimacy of the Party in the villages"*, according to China News Analysis (15 June 1996) No 1562, "Health and Medical Insurance"

On 24 May 2001, Thubten, Head of the TAR Health Department, stated that up to the year 2000 the CMS coverage rate was 1,620,000 persons or 69.8% of the TAR's rural population, 92% in county towns and 89% in townships (Xinhuanet, Tibetinfor.com). The reliability of these statistics is not known; it is clear from reports received by TIN that the degree of implementation of the CMS varies greatly from county to county. There are still many counties in the TAR and in Tibetan areas in Gansu, Qinghai, Sichuan and Yunnan where it is not implemented. There are also great variations in fees to be paid into the scheme.

Just as implementation of the CMS scheme differs from area to area, so does the efficiency of the system in its provision of health care for the poor. In some areas, the costs for joining CMS are said to be reasonable – health workers have quoted examples of 8-15 yuan (US$0.90-1.80) per year in areas of the TAR, which they judge to be affordable for most of the local population. In some areas, very poor people are allowed to defer payment to the CMS or receive free medical care if they persuade the local authorities that they are in need. In others, management of the scheme is reportedly ineffective or corrupt, and some people do not receive adequate medical care even if they have paid into the scheme. Tibetans are sometimes wary about contributing to the system due to mistrust of local officials and concern about the mismanagement of finances.

A recent survey of the CMS system carried out in three counties of Lhasa Municipality by a Western non-governmental organisation (NGO) gave a breakdown of funds provided for CMS by the local authorities. In the areas under study, different levels of government subsidise 15 yuan (US$1.80) to each villager for medical fees; 10 yuan (US$1.20) from the TAR authorities, 3 yuan (US$0.30) from the prefecture and 2 yuan (US$0.24) from the county level. Fees under the CMS in the three counties in the Lhasa area under study represented 1.5% to 3% of a household's total annual income; it is up to the township authorities what percentage is collected – 8 yuan (US$0.90) per person is a common amount. There is provision in some areas to include people within the CMS system without paying any fees – for example, some disabled or infirm elderly people – according to the local health authorities of the three counties.[3]

3 According to official information provided for the study of the CMS system in three TAR counties, the budget of CMS is divided according to the following priorities: 75% of the budget should be spent on costs of out-patient and in-patient treatment, 10% should be used for child immunisation, preventing infectious diseases, maternal and child health care, development of the CMS system, and subsidising village and township health workers who work on prevention activities; another 10% should be used to support in-patients who get serious diseases and households who become poor because of serious or prolonged illness; 3% of the funds should be saved for emergency situations such as the outbreak of unexpected infectious diseases, and 2% of the budget should be spent on CMS's forms, certificates, receipts and annual rewards. Examples of medical treatments that are not reimbursed by CMS in one county include the following: self-poisoning and injury due to vehicle accidents, intoxication or fighting, cosmetic surgery and dental work (for instance the provision of artificial legs and hands, also provision of spectacles), provision of various vitamins and rabies shots or of hepatitis B injections, health check-ups and patient assistance fees, registration fees and medicines bought without a doctor's prescription or authorisation

The same report stated that a management committee formed by the leaders of township governments has the responsibility to manage the budget of CMS involving the collection of money from participants and purchase of medicines for township and village clinics.[4] Participation in CMS in the three counties under the study is up to individual households, according to the report, with the proviso that the participant's *hukou* (Tib: themtho), or household registration, should be in the township where he or she wants to join the CMS. Each member of the household who contributes is given a certificate for future treatment and reimbursement.

A Western health worker who has worked in the TAR told TIN: *"In some areas people have to pay the whole medical fee and then apply for* [their] *refund* [if they have been paying into the CMS]*, and in some areas this application for a refund can only take place on one day of the year or one day every six months or one day every season. In other counties people do not have to pay the full medical fee; they pay for example 30% and the county directly claims the other 70% from the prefecture. The CMS only works where people can afford to pay into the system; if you cannot, you are left without medical care. In parts of China, such as areas in Gansu,* [this] *system has collapsed; poor people go into debt when they are sick if they have not been paying into the system."*

One Western organisation, UNICEF, is making its support of health work in a particular area of Tibet conditional on the county's fair implementation of the CMS system. Another Western NGO based in the TAR has reported the following: *"CMS has improved drug supply and funding of referrals, but still encounters many problems due to the lack of training and understanding from the township authorities. The unspent funds (townships are afraid of running out of money, and do not spend enough, particularly on referrals), might lead the authorities to retain their contribution (the so-called 'free medical care' fund) or to tap CMS to pay for non-government health workers' salaries."*

One of the biggest failings of the CMS system is that it only partially covers fees for hospital admission for a serious illness or surgery. The refund for people attending the village health worker or township clinic for health care is usually around 70%. If the patient is referred to the county hospital, the refund for an out-patient visit is around 35-45% and if they are an in-patient, around 50% of the cost will be reimbursed. However, reimbursement for treatment at the larger prefectural hospital would generally be lower, and the costs higher.

4 According to the report, there is also a CMS monitoring committee, set up to supervise budgets, comprising members from the County People's Congress, the Party Committee, the Commission for Discipline Inspection, the Supervisory Committee and the Village Administration Committee. Township hospitals and village clinics are not included in these two management organisations

A Western health professional told TIN: *"Health care at the village and township level is affordable for most people. What the average person needs is an insurance system that will help them when they require surgery or need long-term specialist treatment for serious illness. The CMS does not help with this because the percentage reimbursed still leaves the person to pay hospital fees that are often exorbitant and unaffordable to most families. A Tibetan family can be ruined financially if just one family member requires hospital admission for a serious illness, accident or surgery."*

A Tibetan official involved in health work in the TAR said: *"If poor people need medical treatment and they are not in the CMS system they need to go into debt. If you are not in the CMS system you should get funds reimbursed from the government but in effect this does not happen. If someone needs a caesarean section, for instance, and they have no money, and are not in the CMS system, they have to sell their animals or they get no care."* The same official said that very poor people had the 'Blue Book' system that entitled them to free medical care, but that this system is being phased out where the CMS is in place. The official added: *"This means that people who are poor and have not paid into CMS have to rely on the compassion of the doctor – maybe the doctor will agree to treat them free of charge."*

If properly implemented, the CMS system should help to resolve some of the basic issues of affordability and equity within the health care service. However, other issues, such as accessibility to medical treatment and health workers' education and training, would have to be addressed as well. Reports from Tibet indicate that just as in rural China, the CMS system does not appear to work effectively to provide adequate health care provision for Tibetans, particularly in rural areas.

Drugs and injections: their cost and use

The CMS system is said to have worked in some ways by expanding the drug supply at township level. However, Western NGO experts who have worked in the TAR report that there are still many problems relating to the procurement and use of available drugs.

One such NGO reported:

> *"The benefit of drugs lies not in the chemical nature of the drug per se, but on the right selection for the particular ailment in correct dosage form at the correct interval and for the correct length of time. Appropriate recommendation of drugs for the patient is vital to achieve the desired effects.*

> *The pharmaceutical need* [in one particular area of the TAR studied] *was determined not on the basis of patient attendance rate, neither from health facility morbidity patterns and standard treatment schedule, but was based on the health workers' understanding of their use. Health workers from township clinics* [in the area] *procured many non-essential drugs including hormones. The management of inventory of drugs stored, expenditure, monitoring, and so on, was non-existent in the clinics. Lastly and more importantly the rationale of prescribing and appropriate dispensing by the health workers was found to be far from satisfactory. Equipment available [in one hospital in the area studied] was found to be lying idle due to lack of training in its use."*

A Western health professional who has worked for several years in the TAR gave TIN the following account of drugs commonly available in township clinics and their use:

> *"People who are not in the CMS system* [in the TAR] *pay 30% more for medications compared with people in the system* [This percentage is likely to vary in different parts of the Tibet]. *Injectable medicines cost much more than oral. There is a usual array of injectable medications in most of the township clinic cupboards. For instance, there are normally boxes of vitamin C. In the West this is rarely injected, and would only be used for severe scurvy (vitamin C deficiency), extensive burns or delayed fracture healing because it stimulates collagen formation and tissue repair) or post-operative wound healing. Usually there are boxes of Gentamycin too. This is an old, cheap, excellent antibiotic that is only available in injectable form. It is a life-saving treatment for very serious infections such as meningitis, endocarditis (infection of the heart muscle) and life-threatening skin infections that are resistant to other antibiotics. However in Tibet (and China) it is cheap, easily available and used unnecessarily for any type of infection, even viral infections. It has many serious side-effects, one of which is deafness (ototoxicity) and toxicity of the kidneys leading to impaired renal function (nephrotoxicity). In the West it has long been replaced by other less toxic drugs. A lot of the deafness in Tibet is attributable to this drug. Unless new, disposable* [sterile] *equipment is used, every injection – whether intramuscular or intravenous – brings with it the risk of blood-borne illness (hepatitis B, C or HIV), paralysis or limping as a result of the wrong technique (for example an injection in the buttock hitting the sciatic nerve) and/or the formation of abscesses as a result of infection. Hepatitis B is very prevalent, far above the average found in China."*[5]

5 A study by one NGO working in the TAR stated that the rate of hepatitis B in the TAR was double the national average for the rest of China

Hospital conditions and neglect of equipment

Tibetans and health professionals working in Tibetan areas frequently refer to the lack of expertise in dealing with medical equipment and the resultant waste of resources, which could frequently be addressed by training programmes.

The following account from a Western aid worker, of their visit to a hospital in the TAR, reflects the standards of health care in hospitals in Tibetan areas generally:

> *"In the county hospital*[6] *the delivery room does not have heating. Low temperatures inside the delivery room, particularly during the winter, may expose new-borns to abrupt cold, often the cause of fatal complications such as hypothermia. Other equipment such as ultrasound, incubators and phototherapy equipment were seen wrapped with clothes. They were lying unused. The doctor told us that different donors without any orientation and training donated equipment and they* [the health workers] *did not know how to use them. During our visits to township clinics, it was observed that no clinics had detergents or soap for cleaning and washing."*

A team from the US charity Kham Aid reported a similar experience when visiting a clinic in the remote county of Nyarong (Chi: Xinlong), Kardze (Chi: Ganzi) Tibetan Autonomous Prefecture (TAP), Sichuan. The Kham Aid team found:

> *"...a startling range of equipment, gastric lavage machine* [for stomach pumping to remove poisons], *oxygen concentrators and abortion machine sitting untouched in a store-room, still in their original packaging. Most local people could not afford or did not understand the need for such services and the doctors did not have the skills to operate the machines."*[7]

6 Exact details of the whereabouts of the hospital have been withheld; it is in a nomadic and farming area of the TAR

7 See the Kham Aid website, www.khamaid.org/ for further information on the charity and the team's assessment of health facilities in an area of Kham (now incorporated into Sichuan province)

Access to affordable health care

> *"Instead of merely throwing money at the problem, training staff on the ground and allowing affordable treatment to the poorer people by means of basic, robust equipment seem to be far more effective. It seems that the existing health system* [in Tibet] *caters only for the newly emerging upper-classes and has forgotten the remaining population, which needs equal priority in all aspects of medicine."*
>
> – a Western student doctor who has worked as a volunteer in the TAR[8]

Reports received by TIN from Tibetans confirm a widespread shortage of affordable and appropriate health care, particularly in rural Tibet. The type of health care on offer is often inappropriate to their needs or of poor quality.[8]

A Western NGO stated after a survey of medical practice in central Tibet:

> *"The main obstacle to health care for villagers was universally identified as cost. It does not matter where they go for treatment, the issue of payment is always a problem. In theory there is a referral system that enables villagers to receive free treatment from their local health worker, and provided they go through each level of the referral system, they should receive free treatment at every level, including the* [local] *City hospital. In practice, however, this system clearly fails... Whether or not the villagers* [in the survey] *are right about having to pay a deposit (and health officials argue they are not right), the fact is this is what they believe. And given that they believe this, it influences how they act in response to illness. Until they are convinced otherwise, their health-seeking behaviours will reflect their attitude to a health system they feel is largely beyond their reach."*

In a December 2001 report to the World Health Organisation (WHO) the Commission on Macro-economics and Health singled out rural western China as one of the main areas in the world where the poor are excluded from 'essential' health care.[9]

8 See the following website: hwww.studentbmj.com/back_issues/0500/life/160.html for an account of the students' work in Tibet

9 The report, entitled "Macroeconomics and Health: Investing in Health for Economic Development", states: *"In most middle-income countries, average health spending per person is already adequate to ensure universal coverage for essential interventions. Yet such coverage does not reach many of the poor. Exclusion is often concentrated by region (eg, rural western China and rural north-east Brazil) or among ethnic and racial minorities."*

A Tibetan from the TAR told TIN: *"The public do not have faith in the doctors in the shang* [township] *hospital. It seems they take a lot of money* [for treatment]." Many Tibetans have reported that sometimes substantial 'security' deposits are required. This money must be paid to hospitals or clinics before patients are admitted, sometimes in addition to medical fees and payment for medicine. A Tibetan woman in her twenties from a farming family in Chamdo (Chi: Changdu) prefecture in the TAR told TIN that sometimes jewellery or other objects were given in lieu of cash as a 'security deposit'. She said: *"Sometimes we [have to give] precious corals and turquoise* [instead of cash] *to the hospital. Later when you give the money they will return these. The hospital staff make profit from the interest on medical fees."* The type of security deposit accepted varies according to the individual hospital or local authority.

A young Tibetan nomad told TIN:

> *"If poor people fall sick they have to borrow money from others and take it to the hospital. Otherwise it seems they cannot keep anything for a security. If you do not have good money with you the doctors do not examine you well. It seems the medical fees are high. Doctors do not come to us* [in the villages and nomadic areas]*; we have to go them* [in the hospitals and clinics]. *When you are bed-ridden in hospital the fees are very high. If a poor person* [who cannot afford medical treatment] *does not get better on his own, he will die."*

A Tibetan female nurse from Tsolho (Chi: Hainan) TAP in Qinghai, who worked in a county hospital before travelling into exile, told TIN that health care in the area suffered because the hospital had to generate thousands of yuan of income every year and went on to outline the approximate costs for health care in the area:

> *"The only income we could generate was through the sales of medicine, which we received for free from the government and which we could sell. We were told* [by the authorities] *that if we didn't reach the goal of money that the hospital had to generate, 200 yuan (US$24) of our salary would be kept by the office. We never reached the target goal so our salary was reduced by this amount. Also because we didn't reach our goal, private clinics in the area were closed. Equipment for the hospital was not provided by the government, our hospital had to buy it. When people come to stay in the hospital they pay 10 yuan (US$1.20) per night per bed, and they have to give 200 yuan (US$24) as a deposit, which they later get back after calculation of the costs. Most nomads can not afford that, so they take medicines from the smaller government clinic in town, and then keep the sick* [members of the family] *in their own houses."*

The right to health

In addition to domestic legislation, China has ratified a number of international human rights treaties recognising the right to health, including the International Covenant on Economic, Social and Cultural Rights (ICESCR), the Convention on the Rights of the Child (CRC), the International Covenant on the Elimination of All Forms of Racial Discrimination (ICERD) and the Convention on the Elimination of All Forms of Discrimination against Women (CEDAW). As the UN Committee on Economic, Social and Cultural Rights defines it, the right to health *"is not to be understood as a right to be healthy. The right to health contains both freedoms and entitlements. The freedoms include the right to control one's health and body, including sexual and reproductive freedom, and the right to be free from interference, such as the right to be free from torture, non-consensual medical treatment and experimentation. By contrast, the entitlements include the right to a system of health protection which provides equality of opportunity for people to enjoy the highest attainable level of health."*

The ICESCR recognises *"the right to the highest attainable standard of physical and mental health"* and in line with this obligates states parties to take steps towards reducing the rates of still birth, infant mortality and promoting the healthy development of the child; improving environmental and industrial hygiene; preventing, treating and controlling epidemic, endemic, occupational or other diseases; and creating conditions which would assure to all medical services and medical attention in the event of sickness (Article 12). The CRC recognises the right of the child to *"the enjoyment of the highest attainable standard of health and to facilities for the treatment of illness and rehabilitation of health. States parties shall strive to ensure that no child is deprived of his or her right of access to such health care services"* (Article 24 (i)).

In addition to provisions similar to the child health provisions of the ICESCR, the CRC also obligates states to *inter alia* ensure the provision of necessary medical assistance and health care to all children with emphasis on the development of primary health care; to combat disease and malnutrition, including within the framework of primary health care, through, *"inter alia, the application of readily available technology and through the provision of adequate nutritious foods and clean drinking water, taking into consideration the dangers and risks of environmental pollution; to ensure appropriate pre-natal and post-natal health care for mothers; to ensure that all segments of society, in particular parents and children, are informed, have access to education and are supported in the use of basic knowledge of child health and nutrition, the advantages of breastfeeding, hygiene and environmental sanitation and the prevention of accidents; and to develop preventive health care, guidance for parents and family planning education and services."*

Health care in Lhasa

Three 5th-year medical students from the University of Leeds in the UK did work placements in Tibet for a Western charity.[10] They gave the following account of their work in Lhasa:

> *"China is now considered the focus of the Communist system since the collapse of the Soviet Union. We therefore imagined a health care system based on universal access and equality for all citizens. It was a surprise that it is in fact* [a completely private system] *where even the most basic investigations and treatments are paid for in cash and on-the-spot. Unconscious patients had their pockets searched for enough money to pay for an X-ray film, or they simply did not receive one at all. The prices of some of these interventions were often in excess of what a rural worker would earn in 6 months, and so many could not afford even the most basic levels of care necessary to keep them alive in the department. Half of doctors' pay comes directly from prescribing and carrying out procedures, and many patients with seemingly trivial illnesses were admitted to the ward at 200 yuan a night (US$24), with intravenous antibiotics at extra cost, which would drain the resources of a family for weeks. This may explain why many Tibetans seek help from traditional herbalists in Lhasa.*
>
> *"The charity initially wanted to supply the hospital with previously lacking reliable water, electricity, and heating supplies, whereas the hospital directors requested 40 ambulances with satellite tracking for Lhasa's 200,000 population, in addition to a computer network and computed tomography*[11] *scanners for the department. The doctor present eventually managed to formulate a plan for an emergency medical care system throughout Tibet, with promises of high-tech equipment to follow at a later stage. When we were there medical equipment worth US$100,000 was delivered to one district hospital to set up an emergency room, which also required painstaking training of the staff in trauma management. In the past, ventilators and high-tech scanning equipment were donated to the hospital by Japanese companies, but the erratic power supply and lack of trained technicians left them collecting dust after a few weeks."*

10 A report on the students' experiences in Tibet is published on the University of Leeds website at: www.studentbmj.com/back_issues/0500/life/160.html

11 Tomography is a method of body imaging in which the X-ray source and/or detection device (e.g. film) rotate around the patient

Tibetan involvement in health projects

A Tibetan with experience of aid projects in Tibet made the following comments on difficulties involved with Tibetan participation in health and education projects in the field:

> *"An official working in Tibet said to me, it's too difficult to have the full involvement of local people in project implementation because generally people* [are supposed to] *think the Party has the perfect solution* [to all problems] *and by emphasising the local people you're undermining the Party. Secondly, because this is a democratic process, by doing this, you're encouraging people to challenge the authorities, which are not democratic. In fact it is vitally important to measure how much the* [foreign] *NGOs involve local participation. As a Tibetan I've been critical of international NGOs – there are some areas where enormous reserves are coming from outside that make people very dependent on the outside organisation and limits their own initiative. I don't want to have this psychology of dependence in my country. My belief is that what's important is not the project but how the project is approached. It's important to allow the people in Tibet to do the project and find the solutions – the project may fail but then a new one can be started with the lessons learnt. Then we're really contributing to the development of a civil society. The best thing is not necessarily to provide a clinic, the best thing is providing education and training to create this clinic, I tell local people it's not the responsibility of the foreign NGO concerned to do this work, it's their responsibility. There are different strategies of local participation – for instance, the county government requests a clinic from an NGO, the NGO asks the local people their opinion, they* [the local people] *laugh, think their opinion is not important. But you explain how important their involvement is going to be in inflencing the result. You don't always have the luxury of dealing on a one-to-one basis, so have to adopt strategies to discuss with a group. In Tibet it takes a long time to really trust people, this creates a barrier, people say to you, I think this, but if you ask me in the meeting I won't tell you, I'll only tell you outside the meeting. It changes their attitude, though, if you say our project includes you, it's your project, it's important to talk in the language of transferring the ownership of the project to locals."*

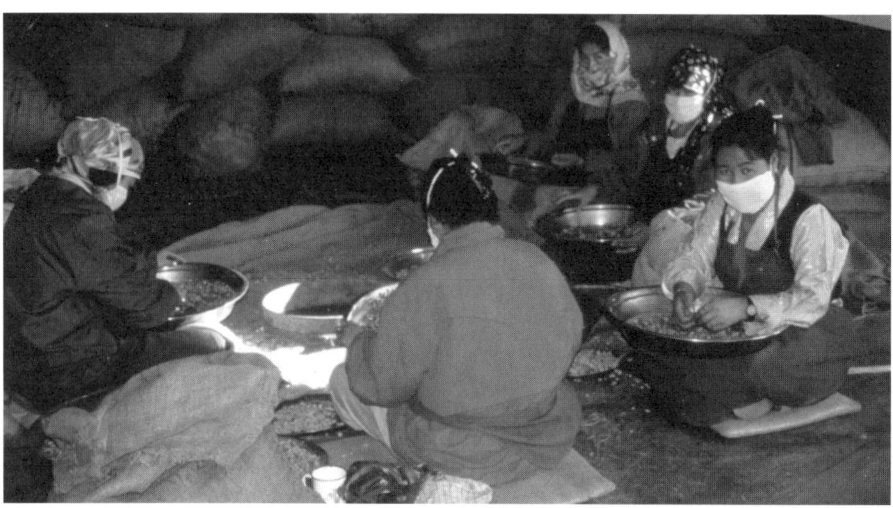

Women preparing ingredients for Tibetan traditional medicine **© Irene Greve/Tibet Images**

Tradition and modernity: Tibetan traditional medicine

For many Tibetans seeking treatment of disease, traditional Tibetan medicine (TTM) (Tib: sorig) offers a comparatively cheap alternative to the western allopathic medicine introduced to Tibet by China. As with the traditional Chinese medicine system (TCM), TTM has remained a 'living tradition', although TTM appears to have been suppressed to a greater extent during the Cultural Revolution. This is primarily due to its roots within the traditional Tibetan religious system.[12] In 'old' Tibet, prior to the Chinese takeover, medical schools were either monasteries or closely related to religious institutions, though there was always a great number of lay *amchis* (Tibetan doctors). It is predominently this lay tradition of TTM that was revitalised in Tibet from the 1980s onwards, under the auspices of the state authorities. TTM has proven effective for the treatment of chronic conditions and relatively benign infections and diseases. In the case of acute infections requiring immediate treatment as well as in the field of surgery, however, the modern school of medicine appears to be more effective when properly practised. This difference is widely acknowledged by the Tibetans who generally adopt a pragmatic approach to the choice of either style of medicine.

12 In 1977, two Chinese authors, His Changhao and Kao Yuanmei, explained that while Tibetan medicine had previously *"been used as a tool to exploit and oppress the working people"*, practitioners were now carrying out research and working on *"the systemisation of Tibetan medicine"* which involved the discarding of *"feudal and superstitious trash"*. From "Tibet Leaps Forward", Beijing, Foreign Languages Press, 1977. TIN thanks Shannon Conrad for highlighting this quote in her final paper on Understanding Modern Tibet, "Traditional Medicine and Ideas of Resistance in Modern Tibet" for Columbia University. See also Craig R Janes, "Tibetan Medicine at the Crossroads: Radical Modernity and the Social Organisation of Traditional Medicine in the TAR, China" in Conner, Linda, and Samuel, Geoffrey, "Healing Powers and Modernity: Traditional Medicine, Shamanism and Science in Asian Societies", Westport, CT: Bergin and Garvey 2000

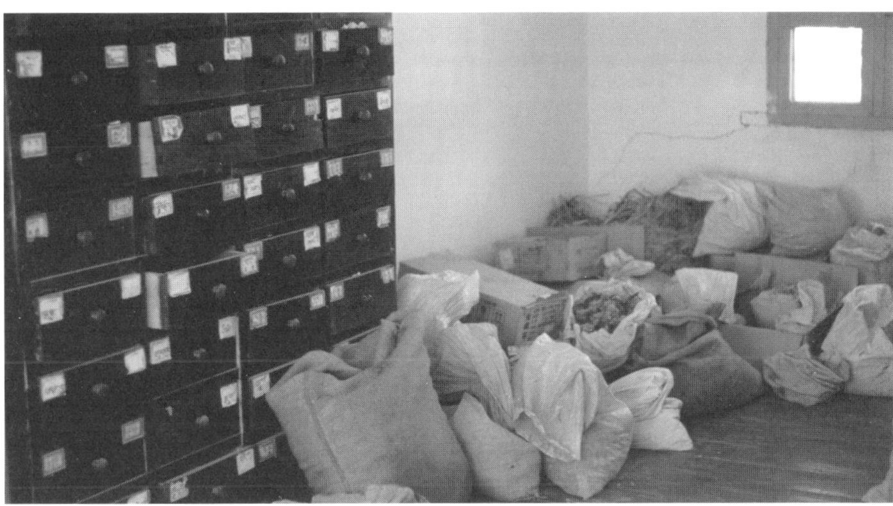

Storeroom for Tibetan traditional medicine © Catherine Platt/Tibet Images

A worldwide demand for TTM, generated mainly by the Tibetan community in exile, has created a growing market for traditional Tibetan medical ingredients from particular plants. It is primarily in response to this development that the commercial cultivation and exploitation of medicinal plants has begun in different Tibetan areas within the PRC, resulting in an emerging state-sponsored industry.[13]

The issue of TTM, its use, development and commercial aspects will be explored in another forthcoming volume of TIN's series on health and health care in Tibet.

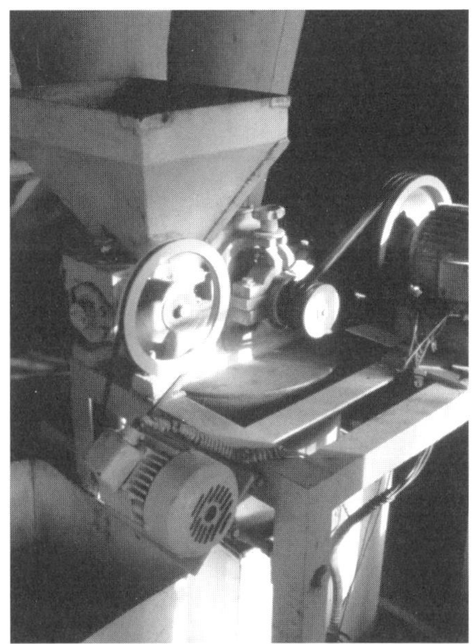

Machine for making TTM pills
© Irene Greve/Tibet Images

13 A recent official publication highlighted the authorities' intention to commercialise TTM: *"[Participants at the 2nd Congress on Tibetan medicine in October 1997 in the TAR] agreed that the production of Tibetan medicine should adapt to the market economic structural reform. While maintaining the characteristics of Tibetan medicine, efforts should be made to combine clinical treatment with scientific research, and combine Tibetan medicine with traditional Chinese medicine and Western medicine. Only in this way can Tibetan medicine develop further"* ("Medicare Service in Tibet" by Zhang Yun, China Intercontinental Press 1999)

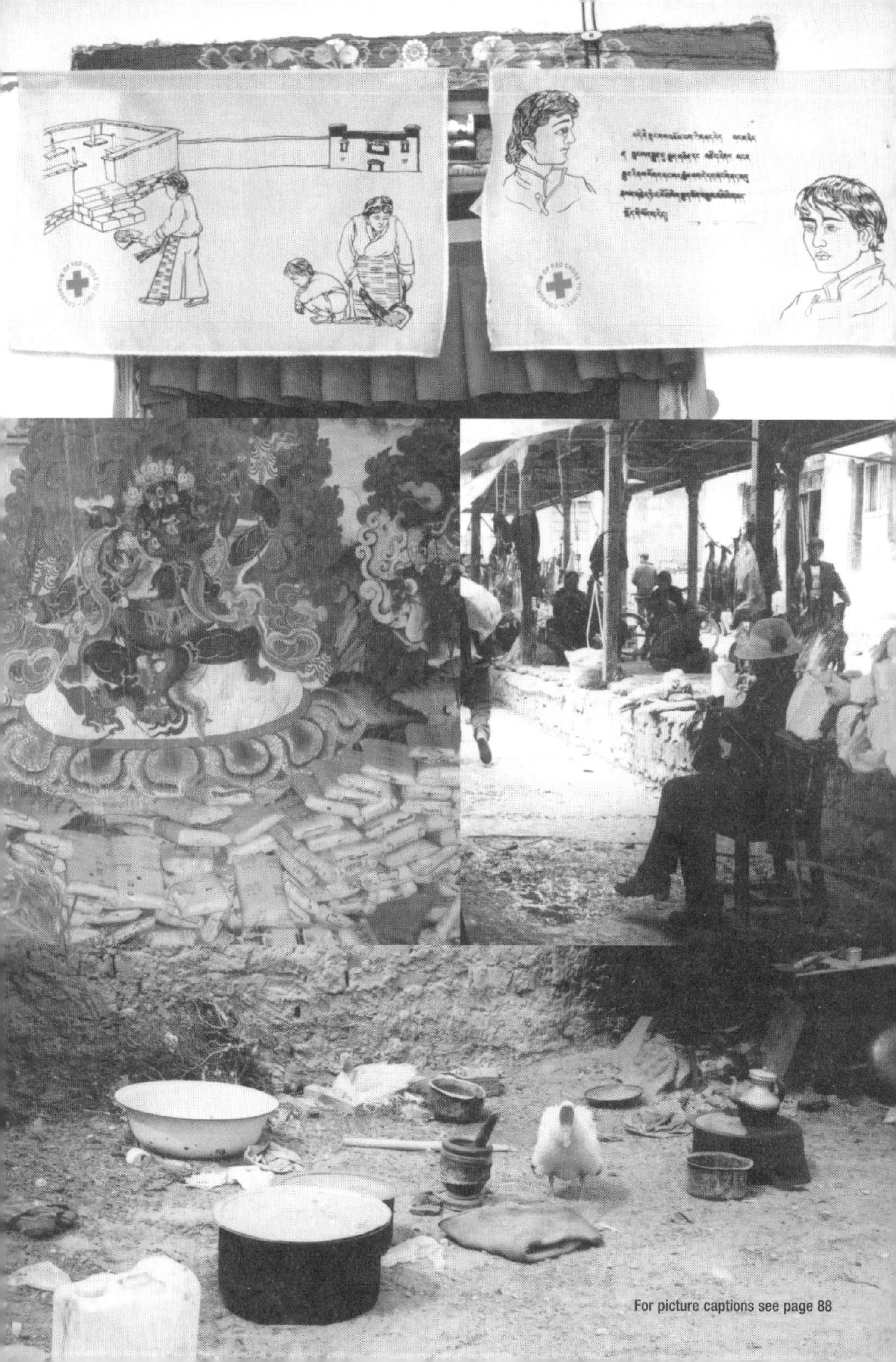

For picture captions see page 88

Chapter Three

Factors affecting health and health care in Tibet

The Tibetan plateau is the highest landmass on earth, with an average altitude of 3,500-5,000m above sea-level, and with the surrounding peaks reaching higher than 7,000m. The climate is extreme, with winter temperatures on the plains plummeting to minus 40 degrees centigrade. Research has shown that Tibetans, in common with other peoples living at high altitudes, have metabolisms that are uniquely adapted to the high altitude of the plateau – they produce higher concentrations of a compound that facilitates oxygen flow throughout the body.[1]

Further studies have confirmed that Tibetans are well adapted physiologically to their high-altitude environment, consistent with their greater generational length of living at a high altitude – they have a larger lung capacity and better maintenance of arterial oxygen saturation during exercise than Chinese acclimatised lowlanders.[2] According to a study on chronic mountain sickness published in 2001,[3] the prevalence of high-altitude heart disease[4] is lower in both sexes of Tibetan high-altitude residents compared with acclimatised newcomers, such as Han Chinese.[5]

People in Tibet reside in widely divergent habitats with varied lifestyles and livelihoods. Health and health care provision is inextricably linked to factors such as the natural resources of the area, including the extent of agricultural land available, animal pasture land, availability of medical herbs, population pressures, and also distances to county seats and large towns.

1 The compound, nitric oxide (NO), is produced in the lungs and helps blood vessels to dilate, thereby allowing oxygen-carrying blood to flow more freely. NO also boosts the oxygen-carrying capacity of haemoglobin, a component of red blood cells. These findings, which are based on a study of people in Bolivia and Tibet, were made by Dr Cynthia M Beall from Case Western Reserve University in Cleveland, Ohio, USA, and colleagues and published in the scientific journal Nature on 22 November 2001

2 Study in Respiration Physiology 1996, Vol 103, Iss 1, pp 75-82: "Smaller alveloar-arterial O-2 gradients in Tibetan than Han residents of Lhasa", Zhuang JG, Droma T, Sutton JR, Groves BM, McCullough RE, McCullough RG, Sun SF, Moore LG

3 "Current concept of chronic mountain sickness: pulmonary hypertension-related high-altitude heart disease", Ge RL; Helun G, Wilderness and Environmental Medicine 2001, Vol 12, Iss 3, pp 190-194.

4 High altitude heart disease is characterised by right ventricular enlargement, pulmonary hypertension and re-modelling of pulmonary arterioles. Most patients have complete recovery on descent to a lower altitude, but symptoms recur with a return to high-altitude

5 Scientists carrying out a study of both Chinese and Tibetan babies born in Lhasa found that Tibetan new-borns had higher arterial oxygen saturation (referring to the amount of oxygen in the blood) at birth and during the first 4 months of life than Han Chinese new-borns, indicating that Tibetans were biologically better-equipped to cope with the high altitudes than the Chinese babies (less oxygen is available to the blood and tissues of the body at a high altitude).
"Arterial oxygen-saturation in Tibetan and Han infants born in Lhasa, Tibet," by Niermeyer S, Yang P, Shanmina, Drolkar; Zhuang JG, Moore LG, published in the New England Journal of Medicine 1995, Vol 333, Iss 19, pp 1248-1252

Changing socio-economic and environmental conditions in many parts of Tibet – resulting in air-bourne pollution, poor hygiene, contaminated water supply and inadequate sewerage systems – are affecting the population in both urban and rural areas. Often these problems occur because of a focus on short-term profit in an environment of rapid modernisation, which frequently leads to the 'cutting of corners' in construction and commercial enterprises, and the neglect of basic facilities, such as sanitation. Issues such as the pollution of water sources can also affect Tibetans living in rural areas, who earn a living from farming, herding or pastoralism. Many of these Tibetans live in areas that are far away from health clinics or hospitals, and when care is needed they have to travel several days by foot or horse to reach the nearest medical facility. Emergency services, even the most rudimentary of facilities, are almost non-existent other than in some major urban centres.

Major health problems in Tibet

> *"The biggest impact on overall health and life expectancy globally has been basic health care and public health interventions to reduce smoking and improve the diet. Facilities such as computed tomography and magnetic resonance image scanning, so sought after in Lhasa, have little impact in a country where most die without ever reaching any hospital or clinic. The hospitals, in trying to catch up with the rest of China, need to have basic hygiene and sanitation inside their buildings and a health policy that tackles the widespread poverty, poor diet, and lifestyle outside."*
>
> – student doctors from the University of Leeds, UK who worked in Tibet[6]

Pulmonary diseases, such as tuberculosis (TB), pneumonia and asthma are widespread in Tibet. Tibet has the highest rate of TB in the PRC[7] (see Chapter Five). Contributory factors include cigarette smoking[8] and a lack of knowledge about the spread of disease, for example the practice of spitting in communal areas. Pneumonia tends to be over-diagnosed in Tibet, while asthma is under-diagnosed – due in part to a lack of understanding coupled with a lack of basic medications to actually treat asthma. Respiratory infections are generally diagnosed as pneumonia, and treated unnecessarily with expensive intravenous antibiotics. Similarly many early cases of lung cancer are not detected, and are instead treated as pneumonia.

6 A report on the students' experiences in Tibet is published on the University of Leeds website at: http://www.studentbmj.com/back_issues/0500/life/160.html

7 Reported by Mary Maish MD, in "Health Care in Tibet: Clinical and Policy Perspectives", Harvard Health Policy Review, Spring 2001 Vol 2, No 1, among other sources

8 There has been an increase in smoking in Tibet – cigarettes are widely available and cheap. China is the world's largest producer and consumer of tobacco, and surveys in the 1990s found that 63% of men and 4% of women were smokers. The 10th World Congress on Tobacco and Health held in Beijing in 1997 reported that about 700,000 people in China died of smoking-related diseases each year. Quoted in "Modern China: A Companion to a Rising Power" by Graham Hutchings, p 183 (Penguin, 2000). The rates of lung cancer in Tibet are likely to rise as the number of smokers increases

Malnutrition and stunting, leading to impaired development, are major problems in Tibet. Recent research showed that the prevalence of stunting due to malnutrition is higher in Tibet than anywhere else in the PRC (see Chapter Five). Tibetan herders often subsist on a diet of meat and barley, with little in the way of vegetables; poor nutrition may also occur when farming households are selling too many of their crops and purchasing less nutritious – but less expensive – substitutes. The incidence of cretinism (retardation of physical and mental development)[9] is high, often due to children being born retarded due to maternal iodine deficiency.

There is a high incidence of rickets (a disorder involving softening and weakening of the bones of children)[10] that is primarily caused by lack of vitamin D or lack of calcium or phosphate. Vitamin D is a fat-soluble vitamin that may be absorbed from the intestines or may be produced by the skin when the skin is exposed to ultraviolet light (particularly sunlight). Although there is a considerable amount of sunshine, Tibetan children are generally kept well wrapped up to protect against the sunburn caused by the high altitude and also the cold weather in the winter months. Deficiency in vitamin C also leads to illness and poor health in Tibetan areas. Vitamin C enhances the absorption of iron, and the risk of mortality in pregnant women during delivery tends to increase in vitamin C deficient populations. Anaemia, a condition when the level of red cells, and therefore of haemoglobin, in the blood is abnormally low, meaning that the oxygen-carrying capacity of blood is reduced, is also common in Tibetan areas and is a risk particularly for women.[11] Anaemia increases the risks of complications during child-birth as well as causing the mother to be less productive economically due to increased tiredness. Breast milk production is adversely affected by anaemia. The mother may fail to pass on sufficient iron stores to her new-born child and therefore unless she feeds iron-rich food as early as the sixth month of life, the child may well become anaemic – meaning that child will be less active, achieve less at school and generally have a slower rate of development.

9 If this condition is left untreated, growth is stunted and the physical stature attained is that of a dwarf. In addition, the skin is thick, flabby, and waxy in colour, the nose is flattened, the abdomen protrudes, and there is a general slowness of movement and speech. If discovered early enough and treated with thyroid extract and sufficient iodine intake throughout life, growth may become normal and mental facility greatly improved. If the condition commences after adulthood is reached it is called myxedema

10 Rickets causes progressive softening and weakening of the bone structure. There is a loss of calcium and phosphate from the bone, which eventually causes destruction of the supportive matrix. The parathyroid gland may increase functioning to compensate for decreased levels of calcium in the bloodstream, resulting in even more loss of calcium and phosphorous as it is reabsorbed from the bones. In severe cases, cysts may develop in the bones. Rickets is most likely to occur during periods of rapid growth where the body demands high levels of calcium and phosphate. It is usually seen in young children from 6 to 24 months old, and is uncommon in new-borns. Rickets is also associated with developmental delays and acute respiratory infection in children

11 Decreased production of red cells is mainly caused by iron deficiency, vitamin B12 deficiency, or folic acid (a vitamin, also called folate) deficiency

Studies show that visual blindness and impairment rates are much higher in Tibet than in comparable communities in mainland China.[12] Other conditions prevalent in Tibet include hepatitis B, Iodine Deficiency Disorders (IDD) (leading to retardation and goitres) and Kashin-Beck (Big Bone) disease – Tibet has one of the highest incidence in the world of this rare disease, which causes retardation, birth deformities and stunted growth (see Chapter Six). The incidence of echinococcosis (also called hydatid disease) – an infection caused by the larvae of the dog tapeworm and transmitted by humans ingesting the faeces of an infected canine – is also of concern to the authorities in Tibet.[13] On 19 September 2002, the Tibet Daily reported that the condition has *"a relatively high rate of incidence in our region amongst the masses in nomadic areas where there is regular contact with goats, cattle and dogs"*. The same report stated that the Lhasa City People's Hospital had cured 119 hydatid disease sufferers, but added that these statistics were 'incomplete'. According to the Chinese authorities, life expectancy in the TAR is 67 years (Xinhua, 8 April 2002) while in China it is 71.8 years (People's Daily, 28 March 2002).

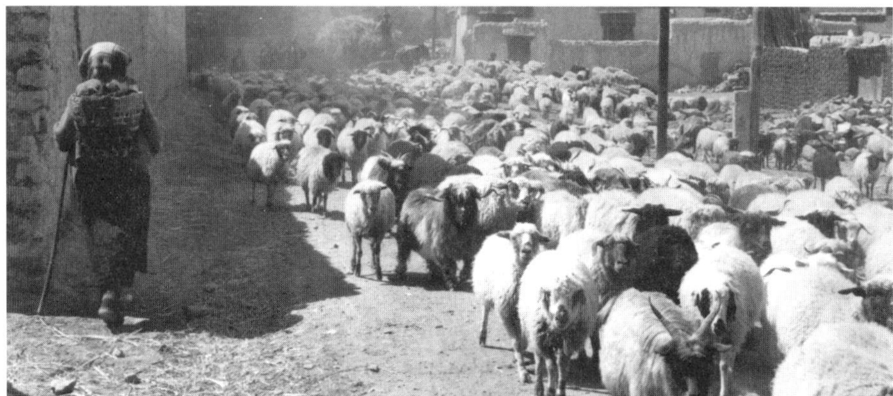

A shepherdess herds her sheep through village in rural Tibet **©Plumpyji/TIN**

12 This may reflect a combination of meteorological (excess ultraviolet irradiation) and nutritional/poverty factors. A study by one group of western health professionals found an extremely small rate of visual impairment in school age children in Tibet; neither trachoma nor vitamin A related blindness were significantly encountered and more than 50% of blindness in the areas under study was due to cataracts

13 Hydatid disease is a parasitic infection by the hydatid larvae (larvae of the dog tapeworm). It is transmitted to humans by the ingestion of food or water contaminated with faeces containing eggs from infected dogs. Once ingested, the eggs hatch and larvae penetrate the intestinal wall and, via the blood stream, travel to and lodge in the liver, lungs, and other organs of the body. Over a number of years the larvae develop into a large, fluid filled sac (hydatid cyst), which contains millions of spores. Large cysts can contain several litres of fluid. As sheep are a common intermediary for the development of the dog tapeworm, hydatid disease is common in sheep-raising countries such as Australia, New Zealand, South Africa, the Middle East and the Mediterranean region. It is thought that most human infections are acquired during childhood and, due to the slow growth of the cyst, symptoms do not appear for decades. In organs, the cysts cause the same symptoms as a solid tumour. As the most common infected organ is the liver, the usual symptoms of infection are abdominal pain, jaundice, and detectable swelling. The cysts can also rupture, causing fever, urticaria (hives), and anaphylactic shock (allergic reaction), and lead to a spread of the larvae and formation of multiple cysts in other organs. Inadequate hygiene practices is one of the main reasons that hydatid disease exists among nomads in Tibet. Fuel is needed to boil water and is scarce in the countryside. Also, if people are too poor to own animals, there is no dung for fuel

Hygiene and its link to health

> "[Our visit to the dentist at the Tibetan hospital] *was like this: all the other patients* [who were waiting to be treated next] *were standing around the patient, then there was a pot with pus and blood standing right next to it, and the doctor just cleaned his bloody drill on his dirty apron which was crusty with blood, and then put it right into the next mouth.* [He] *didn't even disinfect, nothing. He just grubbed around a little bit on the tooth. And then the patient caught an infection, so that he got really high fever. And there is nothing like fillings there; just out with the tooth."*
>
> – a Westerner who has worked in Tibet

> *"After the reform of democracy in Tibet in 1959, Tibet established sanitation and hygiene committees in its cities and counties which helped Tibetan people develop a habit of washing and bathing, encouraged haircuts, eliminated louses and ensured human beings lived apart from domestic animals"*
>
> – Medicare Service in Tibet by Zhang Yun (China Intercontinental Press February 1999)

A lack of education among poorer communities means that people are frequently unaware of issues of nutrition and hygiene, which contributes to sickness and disease. Household hygiene is generally poorly understood; in many rural houses, chickens or other animals have a free run of people's homes and are often seen eating leftover food from cooking utensils used by the family. Food is often left uncovered, which is a problem in summer when the temperature can be quite hot and there are many flies. Tibetans often blow their nose in their hands, and then fling the discharge on the ground inside their home. In it not uncommon or Tibetans to eat old food or bad-smelling meat, and for their drinking water to have not been boiled.

Hygiene practices are dependent on the availability of water and distance to retrieve it – for instance, oral rehydration therapy requires access to 'safe' water and also fuel, so that the water can be boiled (if the water is not properly boiled, the oral rehydration solution can be dangerous, if improperly administered it can aggravate diarrhoea). The fuel needed to boil water is scarce in the countryside; poor families who do not own animals face particular problems if they cannot afford to buy dung to use as fuel.

According to various medical studies, water quantity is often as important as water quality in the prevention of disease, because cleanliness as a result of frequent washing with soap has been shown to reduce ill health. For this reason, many of the Western non-governmental organisations (NGOs) involved in health care in Tibet have prioritised the provision of greatly increased supplies of water to Tibetan villages.

Water supplies can be improved in a relatively cost-effective way by using plastic pipes to bring water from mountain springs into village settlements. This also makes a tremendous difference to the lives of village women, who would otherwise have to spend time and energy in carrying household water for long distances. Time saved can then be spent on other tasks such as childcare, which thus benefits the health of the household. The provision of microbially-safe drinking water to Tibetan settlements significantly reduces the possibilities of drinking water that is potentially contaminated with harmful micro-organisms.

The incidence of respiratory tract infections is partially due to the smokiness of kitchens in Tibetan homes from mud stoves or small metal stoves, which are primarily fuelled by dung. The consistency of the dung fuel causes it to smoulder initially before reaching temperatures high enough to combust. In many cases combustion is incomplete, causing the stoves to emit smoke. When combined with poorly constructed flues, the kitchens become filled with smoke and the ceilings blackened with creosote. In many village homes members of the family sleep in the kitchens; the smoky conditions and residual fumes contribute to the inflammation of respiratory tract membranes.

Nutrition, dietary practices and sustainability

Nutritional specialists point out that the diet of Tibetans is adapted to their specific high altitude environment and harsh climate. A western health worker and specialist in nutrition told TIN: "*The Chinese claim that the Tibetan traditional diet is not diverse enough and doesn't provide all the nutrients that are needed. But Tibetans have survived for centuries on their diet and on the whole it is appropriate for the geographical and climatic conditions. Barley, the traditional staple of the Tibetan diet, is one of the most nutritious grains; yak meat is one of the most nutritious of meats, turnips are a good source of vitamin C, beans and milk give protein and butter provides essential fats. The question is what is sustainable, and often these food sources are not adequately available to Tibetans due to the changing nature of life in Tibet. For instance, the Chinese do not want to grow barley, they want to grow wheat, so often cultivation now is focused on wheat, which is not as durable as barley. If there is a drought the wheat will die while barley is more tolerant.*" Similarly, rice is thought to be 'modern' and now Tibetans who have access to purchasing rice will eat it in place of *tsampa* (roasted barley flour), a Tibetan staple. Unlike *tsampa*, white rice has little nutritional value.

The most typical Tibetan foods are *tsampa* and buttered tea. In Tibetan villages, *tsampa* is often the main ingredient of all meals every day throughout the year. It is usually mixed with salted buttered tea to form a thick paste, and when available, extra yak butter is added. In more affluent households the diet is more varied and typically includes dried yak or sheep meat. Animals are usually killed in the early winter and the meat is hung to freeze dry in a shaded place. During the summer families with more resources can also eat a limited number of vegetables such as cabbage, peas, radishes and potatoes. Many health problems in Tibet linked to nutrition occur because of changes in land-use and the various aspects of modernisation in Tibetan areas; families are often unable to grow or purchase sufficient food to provide for their needs (see Chapter Four for an assessment of poverty in Tibetan areas and its link to malnutrition[14]). The details of common health problems presented earlier in this chapter give an indication of widespread deficiencies in the average diet.

One of the most effective ways of improving the lives of people in poor areas is to improve nutrition, according to a set of principles approved by the World Health Organisation (WHO) known as Integrated Management of Childhood Illness (IMCI). IMCI is an integrated approach to child health that takes into account the variety of factors that put children at serious risk. It ensures the combined treatment of the major childhood illnesses, by emphasising the prevention of disease through improved nutrition and immunisation, among other factors.[15] Introducing and implementing the IMCI strategy in any country is a phased process that requires a great deal of co-ordination among existing health programmes and services. According to the WHO, the programme is only in an early stage of implementation in China. The United Nations Children's Fund (UNICEF) has been involved in pilot projects involving the design and management of IMCI programmes in Tibet. UNICEF found that oral rehydration, effective nutritional counselling and nutritional management of persistent diarrhoea are not available to most mothers seeking care for their children in Tibet, and that further training is needed to prepare health workers to deliver nutrition counselling and other preventive health care.

14 An exploration of the issue of land use, the developing economy and food shortages in Tibetan areas is beyond the scope of this report. A conceptual global analysis of this issue is provided in the works of economist Amartya Sen, who has written on the links between food supply, poverty, deprivation, population and entitlements in relation to food shortages and famines, stating that malnourishment frequently results from political and economic iniquities. Sen's work explores the factors that determine the distribution of food within the community. Amartya Sen's 'entitlement approach' concentrates on the ability of the people to command food through the legal means available in society, including the use of production possibilities, trade opportunities, rights vis-à-vis the state and other methods of acquiring food. A person starves because he does not have the ability to command enough food. This 'entitlement approach' concentrates only on those means of commanding food that are legitimised by the legal system in operation in that society. See http://top-biography.com/0036-Amartya%20Sen/works.htm for a summary of the entitlement approach in relation to food shortages

15 According to WHO, IMCI is a set of principles that aim to reduce death, illness and disability and to promote improved growth and development among children under five years of age. IMCI includes both preventive and curative elements that are implemented by families and communities as well as health facilities. For further details see the WHO website at: http://www.who.int/child-adolescent-health/integr.htm

According to one Western representative of an NGO working in Tibetan areas, health workers in the Tibetan health care system do not have any training in nutrition, and rarely make the link between nutrition and health. Pregnant women and children are rarely weighed or measured – weighing scales are mainly unavailable in township clinics. Teachers in the many boarding schools in the TAR will typically have little knowledge of nutrition. In one school where children were weighed and measured by a NGO, chronic malnutrition was found to affect over 50% of children aged between 5 and 12 years.

Micro-nutrient deficiencies appear to vary within Tibet and by season, given the diverse geographical regions and subsistence lifestyles of the Tibetan population, that is, nomadic, semi-nomad, farming and urban, and the harsh winter. Socio-cultural factors play an important role. For example, in the nomadic area of Nagchu (Chi: Naqu) in the TAR, young children are given meat, dairy products and *tsampa*. but often do not obtain enough vitamin C, due to the lack of vegetables at certain times of the year.[16]

A Tibetan from a farming village near Labrang (Chi: Xiahe) in Kanlho (Chi: Gannan) Tibetan Autonomous Prefecture in Gansu province gave TIN the following account of his diet when growing up, and perceptions of food and nutrition among Tibetans:

> *"We didn't normally have fruit to eat, but my father used to go to the TAR on business and he would bring back some fruit as a present because they were sweet and tasty to eat. Otherwise we didn't have a habit of perceiving fruit as healthy and eating it for that reason. We used spinach, white radish, green onion, cabbage and potatoes from our own vegetable garden. Small children were given bread soaked in milk. The nomads would consider our diet not to be very healthy because we didn't have so much meat and butter. They would look at us as though we were eating like Chinese because we ate vegetables. But we did consider meat to be a good food, although we didn't eat as much as the nomads because we didn't have animals. We used to take our own food to school, and in the beginning I would carry tsampa mixed with some butter, dried cheese and the sour liquid that is left from the milk after you have made butter.[17] But then taking tsampa to school became embarrassing because many of the other children were taking home-made bread, and this was regarded as much better."*[18]

16 The Chinese press frequently refers to the 'backward' and 'superstitious' beliefs and habits of Tibetans, and has linked these to their dietary habits. An article in China's Tibet, published on the official website tibetinfor.com on 11 October 2002, presented the rather dubious viewpoint that the changes in the diet of Tibetans is an indictor of *"a kind of psychological emancipation of trans-century significance for Tibetan society."* The article stated: *"Under the impact of social modernisation in the past two decades or so, there have been big changes in the diet of the Tibetan race. Educated people of the young generation agree that all food that is not poisonous is edible. They see no taboos. Under their 'leadership', Tibetans no longer seek a final say from Buddha in the selection of food"*

17 This is likely to be the whey

18 In this particular area, which is populated by many Chinese migrants as well as Tibetans, *tsampa* is associated with poverty and low social status

There are some relatively simple ways of improving basic nutrition for poor Tibetan households, particularly when fruit and vegetables are scarce, although health professionals stress the need to gather information locally before developing feeding recommendations due to the regional variation in lifestyle and dietary practices.

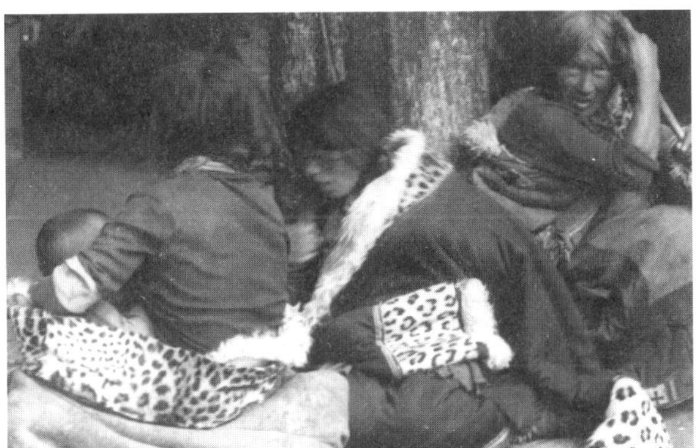

Tibetan women caring for young child **©TIN**

Health workers and nutritionists working in various areas of the TAR have encouraged Tibetan mothers in their habit of adding various various ingredients to *tsampa*, such as extra butter, mashed potatoes, radish, green vegetables, buttermilk, yoghurt, egg, small pieces of meat, dried ground peas, making it into a nutrient-dense porridge. A pinch of iodine salt to *tsampa* fed to babies is also recommended to help prevent goitres, and essential fatty acids can be provided by adding butter or rapeseed oil. Western health care workers in Tibet have also recommended that children from between the ages of 2 and 5 years are given snacks in addition to three meals a day – such as popped barley kernels and roasted peas; glass of buttermilk; nuts and seeds – in order to add essential micronutrients to the diet. In some areas, families believe it is not appropriate to give vegetables to children under the age of 5 years, and in some nomadic areas meat is not given until the children have teeth. UNICEF staff recommend that cooked dark green leafy vegetables, such as nettles, which are commonly available in many areas, are given to young children either mixed with *tsampa* or cooked in a thick soup.

Cultural concerns about vegetables that need to be taken into account by health workers in the field include the wide-spread belief that vegetables are a 'cold food' that cause diarrhoea. There is also the perception in some areas that leafy green vegetables and stinging nettles are perceived as food for animals; at best nettles are perceived as being food for people of low social status or the poor.

19 (see next page) Some Tibetan mothers who have to go out to the fields soon after the birth start to add animal milk and watery gruel to their infants' diets within the first few weeks of age. This appears to be less of a problem for nomadic women, who often breast-feed their children exclusively during the first year

A Western health worker, who has many years of experience working in Tibet, gave TIN the following account of the link between cultural factors, nutrition and the health of Tibetan children:

> *"The World Health Organisation says that babies should be 6 months [old] before eating solids, or before if he or she seems hungry and not satiated by breast-milk. But some Tibetan mothers give their babies tsampa when they are only a month old. This is generally because in nomad and farming families the mothers often have to go out to work in the fields soon after the birth, and so babies are left with the grandmother. Of course the grandmother can't do the breast-feeding, generally, and will often give the baby what other people are eating such as tsampa which doesn't really give them the nutrients they need.*[19]
>
> *While western NGOs encourage Tibetan women to breast-feed, a new type of problem that appears to be emerging in some urban Tibetan areas is that urban Chinese women look down on breast-feeding, and this attitude is spreading to Tibetans. Some Tibetan women feel that it is not enough to give babies breast-milk and so they give them tsampa too, when the baby is too young for solids. Another problem is that tsampa is so bulky that by the time the baby's eaten the tsampa they're too full to drink the breast-milk.*
>
> *The diet of children often becomes worse as they become urbanised, they eat more sugar, and there is a type of Chinese* [white] *bread that has virtually no nutrients at all.*
>
> *Butter is very expensive in many areas. There are different grades, some will mix dri (a female yak) butter with oil, but Tibetans can always tell good butter by the taste. The increase in the price of butter has been phenomenal, so people often can't afford it. You can always tell the level of poverty of a Tibetan household by what they serve as tea. If tea is served with just salt that means they can't afford butter – it is a sign of honour and prestige to give your guests butter tea*[20]*. Butter is ideal for health in terms of the high altitude of Tibet; it's high in calories, you need more calories to keep you warm.*
>
> *Often in farms they'll feed beans to the animals, they feel they're not good enough for humans but will give them as protein to animals. Nomads have a very high protein diet because of milk products from animals. If they lose their herds, nomads have lost everything."*

19 See footnote on previous page

20 Reports from Western visitors to central Tibetan areas frequently bear out the view that even when the household is very poor, Tibetans will still make great efforts to serve butter tea. In the Tibetan traditional area of Kham, even though nomads often have plenty of butter, their preference is black tea with salt and no butter

The lack of education about the factors affecting health

In Tibet, knowledge about the link between food and ill-health, and about hygiene as a cause of disease, is poor among the majority of the population. A Western NGO carried out a survey among villagers in central Tibet about perceptions of health care and what they would do in medical emergencies.

While many of the answers reflected difficulties in access to hospitals and medical facilities (see Chapter Two), most of them indicated a general lack of awareness and education about health care.

For instance, in response to a question about action to be taken when a woman was experiencing problems in giving birth, villagers in one particular area recommended that the first priority should be to give particular types of food to the woman, rather than being taken immediately to a hospital or seeking the advice of a doctor.[21]

The responses also reflect an awareness of poor medical facilities in the area, and appear to be based on the assumption that women will be giving birth at home without proper medical supervision rather than in hospital, which is another issue of concern to health workers in Tibetan areas. One of the responses stated that when difficulties occurred during labour the woman should: *"(1) eat eggs (2) drink bone soup and (3) mix ginger with butter or fresh chang (Tibetan barley beer) and drink it."*

Another response indicated a distinction between poorer standards of health care in villages and in urban areas, stating the following: *"When a family is in good financial shape the woman can go to the hospital. In the village, the woman may be given the following: caterpillar fungus* [yartsa gumba, meaning 'summer grass, winter worm'], *fresh meat, butter and bone soup".*

21 In the West, women are told not to eat during labour, in case they need to have pain-relief

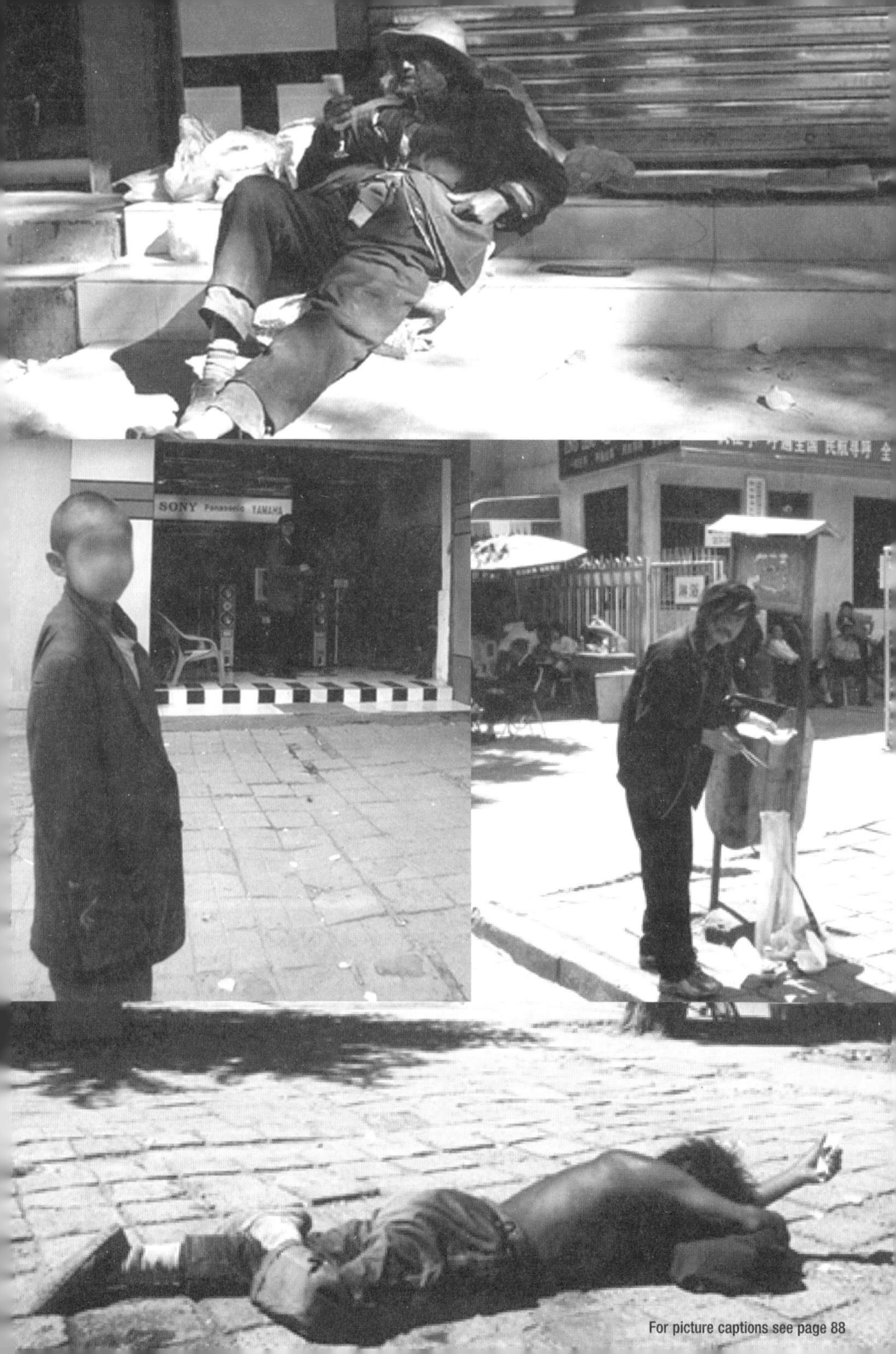

For picture captions see page 88

Chapter Four

Poverty and health

> *"Health is the basis for job productivity, the capacity to learn in school and the capability to grow intellectually, physically and emotionally. In economic terms, health and education are the two cornerstones of human capital, which Nobel* [Economics] *Laureates Theodore Shultz and Gary Becker have demonstrated to be the basis of an individual's economic productivity. As with the economic well-being of individual households, good population health is a critical input into poverty reduction, economic growth, and long-term economic development at the scale of whole societies... Societies with a heavy burden of disease tend to experience a multiplicity of severe impediments to economic progress."*
>
> – Macroeconomics and Health: Investing in Health for Economic Development, Report of the Commission on Macroeconomics and Health[1]

Poverty is a feature of both urban and rural Tibetan society. A health worker with experience in Tibet made the following comment after seeing a severely malnourished child in the centre of Lhasa:

> "[Tibetan] *babies are totally wrapped, [often] in ten layers. If you don't unwrap the child you don't see the pot-bellies and skeletal frames. We saw a child, the size of a newborn child – no teeth, couldn't sit up, your classic African marasmus case.*[2] *The mother was feeding the baby only powdered milk from 2 weeks of age. It was in the Barkor. The eyes are vital* [in terms of diagnosing malnutrition]. *If you can see marasmus in downtown Lhasa, you can imagine what it's like elsewhere."*

1 Presented by Jeffrey D Sachs, Chair, to Gro Harlem Brundtland, Director-General of the World Health Organisation (WHO) on 20 December 2001

2 a severe form of malnutrition and progressive emaciation usually occurring in young children caused by an inadequate intake of both protein and calories

3 (see next page) The goal of promoting primary health care in rural areas is to give basic medical services to every resident, Ministry of Health official Zhang Chaoyang said in an article in People's Daily on 11 June 2002, adding that it *"means a fair society"* Zhang noted that the work was also vital for the global fulfilment of a health-for-all goal set by the WHO

4 (see next page) Paper by Liu Yuanli, a Harvard School of Public Health professor and Rao Keqin, Director of the Ministry of Health's Centre for Health Statistics and Information, funded by the Asian Development Bank and China's State Development and Planning Commission, quoted in "The Sickness Trap" by Susan V Lawrence, the Far Eastern Economic Review, 13 June 2002

5 (see next page) One example of this discrepancy is that 80% of pregnant women in eastern rural areas were expected to deliver babies in hospitals, 60% in central provinces, but only 50% in western regions. In the TAR, women are so frequently living in areas far away from hospitals that it is more of a priority to provide trained health care professionals who can assist them during labour at home if necessary. Research by one NGO in the TAR found that from a sample survey of village women, only 6% of women who gave birth in a 12-month period were attended by someone trained in clean and safe deliveries (see Chapter Five)

The east-west divide

In summer 2002, Beijing policy-makers announced that they were formulating a plan to provide basic health care to 900 million rural residents by 2010 as part of the 'global fulfilment' of the 'health for all' policy of the World Health Organisation (WHO).[3] The ambitious plans, which are probably the first outline of policy to be presented by China to the WHO, aim to make health services accessible to all rural residents, who make up a majority of its population.

International health experts acknowledged the significance of the document – which was produced at a high-level meeting in Beijing, involving seven ministries including the planning and finance ministries – but questioned whether China could deliver on its ambitious proposals, given the current state of health care in the People's Republic of China (PRC), and the fact that state spending on health care in proportion to other services has decreased since the late 1970s.[4]

Beijing acknowledges in the policy outline presented to the WHO the vast discrepancies in provision of health care between eastern and western China. The regional variations in the latest "Outline for the Development of Primary Health Care in Rural Areas of China" are dramatic, with substantial differences in indicators for improvement in health between the eastern and western areas of the PRC, including Tibet.[5]

Not only is there a marked difference between the levels of health care and health indicators in east and west China, there is also a notable divergence between the health of Tibetan people in Tibetan areas compared to the other, poorer, western provinces of China. Assessed in accordance with the Human Development Index (HDI) of the United Nations Development Programme (UNDP) – which takes into account factors including life expectancy, literacy, and infant mortality – the Tibet Autonomous Region (TAR) would have had the lowest HDI ranking of all the provinces in China in both 1990 and 1997, well below even the next ranking provinces of Guizhou and Qinghai in 1997.[6] While China was ranked 98th, the TAR would have ranked 148th, between Madagascar and Yemen, in 1997. This was because the health and education indicators of Tibet were so poor that they pulled the HDI of Tibet far below the level of even the poorest regions of China.[7]

3, 4 & 5 See footnotes on previous page

6 The HDI is an index that aggregates the purchasing price parity GDP per capita with a gross index of life expectancy, approximating health, and education standards. The index is measured on a percentile basis, with the highest possible score being one. If wealth brings about a correspondent level of social development, the HDI ranking should be similar to its GDP per capita ranking. This summary of HDI ranking and assessment of the TAR's ranking is from "Poverty by Design: The Economics of Discrimination in Tibet" by Andrew Fischer, and is published by the Canada Tibet Committee, an independent NGO. To download a copy of the report, published in August 2002, see the Canada Tibet Committee website at: www.tibet.ca/english/index.html

7 See "Poverty by Design", cited above

Poverty, health and development

> *"Health should be seen as an integral part of the development agenda. There is, first of all, the basic recognition that deprivation of health is an aspect of under-development. Just as for the individual, not having medical treatment for curable ailments constitutes poverty, similarly, for a country, not having adequate health arrangements is a part of under-development. So you have to place the issue of health care right at the centre of the development agenda. Secondly, there are enormous inter-dependencies between different kinds of deprivations. For example, the deprivation of health is bad even for the economy because people's productivity depends on their level of nutrition and health."*
>
> – Amartya Sen, Nobel Prize-winning economist[8]

Current economic policy in Tibet is dominated by the authorities' ambitious plans to develop the western regions of China.[9] These plans have evolved due to the political, strategic and economic concerns of the central government rather than the promotion of sustained and integrated local development in Tibetan areas.[10]

Official statistics recording increases in the income of Tibetans and the provision of subsidies for the TAR are misleading, as they do not give a balanced account of the overall economy. Tibet's natural and mineral resources are claimed by the Chinese state, as permitted by Article 9 of the Chinese Constitution. However official statistics do not take into account the value of these resources or much of the agricultural produce sold to the government at fixed rates.

Andrew Fischer, a development economist, writes in his report: "Poverty by Design: The Economics of Discrimination in Tibet":[11] *"Within the recent Chinese government statistics for the* [TAR], *it is actually possible to identify a clear trend towards the marginalisation of ethnic Tibetans within both the national economy and the poorer western regions of China. Although the provincial economy of Tibet (TAR) presumably grew faster than the national Chinese economy throughout most of the 1990s, this growth occurred* [mainly] *in areas that were not accessible to the large majority of ethnic Tibetans, who nonetheless accounted for most of the provincial population.*

8 Quoted in an interview for "To Our Health", the internal newsletter of the WHO, which can be downloaded at: www.who.int/infwha52/to_our_health/amartya.html

9 See the TIN publication "China's Great Leap West", published by TIN in November 2000. For a map of China's western regions see TIN's website at: www.tibetinfo.co.uk/publications/bbp/map_china_western_region.htm

10 See the following website for a copy of Tibetan government in exile guidelines for sustainable development in Tibet in a report presented to the United Nations World Summit on Sustainable Development in 2002: www.phayul.com/sub/wssd/shadow.aspx

11 Andrew Fischer in "Poverty by Design", as above

12 According to the 1999 TAR Statistical Yearbook, which gives figures for 1998, average annual per capita income in the TAR, in rural areas, was 1,590.92 yuan (US$192) and in TAR urban areas was 6,922.56 yuan (US$836)

Meanwhile, the real incomes of most Tibetan people actually fell in the first part of the 1990s, and overall remained stagnant throughout the decade." Fischer reports that the actual purchasing power of the average Tibetan decreased sharply in the first years of the 1990s, although it had returned to the 1990 level by 2000. In 1998, rural incomes in the TAR had become the lowest of all rural incomes in China.[12] The contrasting increase in urban household incomes in the TAR – which indicates one of the highest urban-rural inequalities in China – reflects, in part, the influx of Chinese migrants to the TAR.[13] Economic growth in the TAR has been almost entirely concentrated in the urban industrial and service sectors and has therefore not benefited most Tibetans, who mainly live in rural areas.[14]

The United Nations Committee on Economic, Social and Cultural Rights has defined poverty as *"a human condition characterized by the sustained or chronic deprivation of the resources, capabilities, choices, security and power necessary for the enjoyment of an adequate standard of living and other civil, cultural, economic, political and social rights."*[15]

Amartya Sen, the Nobel Prize-winning economist known for his pioneering work on development in relation to food shortages, inequality and human rights, has described poverty further in the context of geographical, biological and social factors that amplify or reduce the impact of income on each individual. He refers to the interconnectedness of social conditions with poverty, stating that the poor generally lack a number of elements, such as education, access to land, health and longevity, justice, family and community support, credit and other productive resources, a voice in institutions, and access to opportunity.[16]

Sen writes:

> *"If we think of poverty as basic deprivation of the quality of life and of elementary freedoms, then ill-health is an aspect of poverty. Bad health is constitutive of poverty. Premature mortality, avoidable illness, under-nourishment are all manifestations of poverty. I believe that health deprivation is really the most central aspect of poverty."*[17]

13 Andrew Fischer writes: *"For all intents and purposes, [the situation in Tibet] is a socio-economic description of an ethnically distinct, exploited peripheral region controlled from the outside"*. Fischer presents the following suggestions for a policy approach that considers the welfare of the average Tibetan: (i) focus on intensive rather than extensive models of regional development (ii) include strategies to cultivate skills within the indigenous population (iii) develop non-farm rural industries (iv) establish local linkages between farm and non-farm activities (v) prioritise the extension of low-cost, low-tech infrastructure and services

14 China has acknowledged the substantial urban-rural income gap throughout China. China State Statistics Bureau Deputy Director Qi Xiaohua stated that the gap between urban and rural incomes in China is much greater than the 3:1 ratio indicated in official statistics – he admitted that the real gap should be in the ratio of 5:1 or even 6:1 (report by Zhongguo Xinwen She, 21/10/02)

15, 16 & 17 See footnotes on next page

Poor health and disease are both a cause and a consequence of poverty. The poor are much more susceptible to disease due to a lack of access to clean water and sanitation, safe housing, medical care, information about preventive health care and adequate nutrition. As this report has shown, Tibetans in poor communities are often less likely to seek medical care even when it is urgently needed, because of a lack of access to doctors, clinics and hospitals, a lack of resources needed to cover treatment and a lack of knowledge on how to respond to various illnesses. Fees for treatment of serious disease or illness can push people deeper into the poverty trap – from which it is difficult for them to recover – by forcing them into debt, or the sale or mortgaging of assets, such as their land, livestock or homes.

All of these factors are evident in both China and Tibet.[18] The high cost of medical treatment throughout the PRC is contributing to rural poverty, where the poor state of health of Tibetans and Chinese households living below the poverty line is inextricably linked to an inadequate diet, lack of basic facilities and sanitation, resulting in conditions such as malnutrition, stunting, rickets, anaemia, gastro-intestinal problems diarrhoea, parasites, chronic respiratory infection and Iodine Deficiency Diseases.

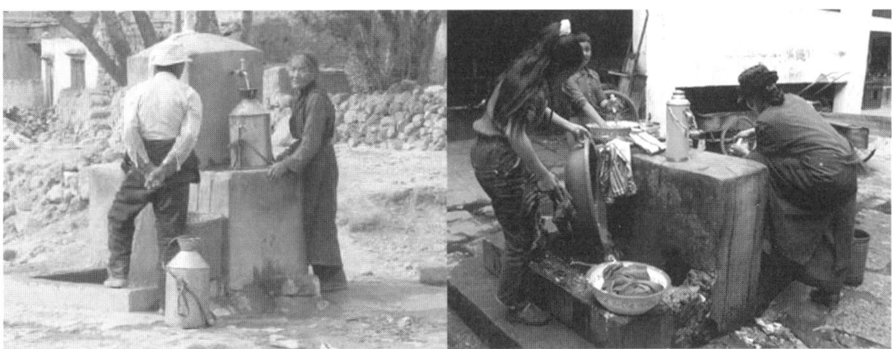

LEFT **a new tap stand in a Tibetan village** **©TIN**
RIGHT **typical communal washing area in urban Tibet** **© Barefoot Images**

15 (see previous page) See the UN Office of the High Commissioner for Human Rights website at: www.unhchr.ch/development/poverty-02.html
16 (see previous page) A summary of Amartya Sen's views on poverty can be downloaded from the Magazine of the Inter-American Development Bank at: www.globalpolicy.org/socecon/develop/2001/1205sen.htm
17 (see previous page) Quoted in an interview for "To Our Health", the internal newsletter of the WHO, which can be downloaded at: www.who.int/infwha52/to_our_health/amartya.html
18 It is worth noting that China has a different, lower measure of poverty than the international community, which must be taken into account when assessing official statistics on poverty alleviation. The measure for absolute poverty in the 9th Five-Year Plan was set at 500 yuan per year in 1990 prices, equivalent to 1,012 yuan (US$122) per year in 1998 prices, or 33 US cents per day (non-purchasing power parity). The World Bank and the Millennium Development Goals set by the international community have all agreed on one US dollar per day (purchasing power parity) as a basic international benchmark for extreme poverty

Health in a macroeconomic context

Countries with poor health care and a high incidence of illness or disease face difficulties in achieving sustained growth. Disease impedes development as a consequence of (i) avoidable disease reducing life expectancy, as well as the annual incomes of individuals and the community as a whole, thereby adversely affecting the prospects for economic growth. (ii) The effects of disease on the returns to business and infrastructure investment, beyond the effects on individual worker productivity, are such that whole industries are undermined by a high prevalence of disease. (iii) The effect of disease on parental investments in children can be that societies with high rates of infant and child mortality have higher birth rates ('fertility rate'[19]) in part to compensate for the frequent deaths of children. This reduces the ability of poor families to invest in the health and education of individual children. Evidence presented by the Commission on Macroeconomics and Health to the WHO[20] showed that in a given time period, countries with lower infant mortality rates experienced higher economic growth during that period.[21]

An effective health strategy should incorporate investments in poverty reduction beyond, but in co-ordination with, the formal health sector, for example in education, water and sanitation, and in the context of Tibet, agricultural improvement. Underlying these investments are broader issues of governance, political aims within a region and the relative importance of development and poverty reduction in national priorities. Health professionals with experience in Tibet confirm that development efforts have: a relatively short time-frame; are characterised by competition rather than collaboration; fail to draw on the accumulated wisdom of the local people as an input; and do not invest significant resources on expanding the capacity of the local people to sustain such development initiatives. There is increasing recognition at the international level that effective poverty reduction is enhanced by the enjoyment of a broad range of human rights.[22]

19 A fertility rate is the measure of fertility (births) among the females of a population. The general fertility rate measures the fertility among women of child-bearing age, and is calculated as the total number of births per 1,000 females ages 15-44 in the population. An age-specific fertility rate is the number of births per 1,000 females in a specified age group. A birth rate is the number of births that occur within a certain population (or area) over a specified time period in relation to the total population of the area. Specifically, it is the number of births per 1,000 total population

20 "Macroeconomics and Health: Investing in Health for Economic Development", Report of the Commission on Macroeconomics and Health, Presented by Jeffrey D Sachs, Chair to Gro Harlem Brundtland, WHO, 20 December 2001. A copy of the report can be downloaded at: www.cid.harvard.edu/cidcmh/CMHReport.pdf

21 A typical statistical estimate presented in the report suggests that each 10% improvement in life expectancy at birth is associated with a rise in economic growth of at least 0.3-0.4% per year

22 For instance, if the poor are to enjoy the right to participate in poverty reduction strategies, they must be free to organise without restriction (right of association), to meet without impediment (right of assembly), and to say what they want without intimidation (freedom of expression); they must know the relevant facts (right to information) and they must enjoy an elementary level of economic security and well-being (right to a reasonable standard of living and associated rights). See: "Draft Guidelines: A Human Rights Approach to Poverty Reduction Strategies", the United Nations Office of the High Commissioner for Human Rights at: www.unhchr.ch/development/povertyfinal.html

The eradication of disease

The Commission on Macroeconomics and Health[23] states that the health prospects of the poorest billion people in the world could be radically improved by targeting a relatively small set of diseases and conditions. The primary targets are as follows: HIV/AIDS, malaria, tuberculosis (TB), maternal and peri-natal conditions, widespread causes of child mortality including Measles, Tetanus, Diphtheria, acute respiratory infection and diarrhoeal disease, malnutrition that exacerbates those diseases, other vaccine-preventable illness and tobacco-related disease. Examples of the incidence of such conditions in Tibet are given below, and in Chapters Three, Five and Six.

Malnutrition and stunting

> *"The children of Tibet are suffering from a silent calamity that causes many to die and that inhibits the development of the survivors. This calamity will have a negative effect on the people of Tibet for generations to come."*
> – Glen E Maberly and Kevin M Sullivan, New England Journal of Medicine, 01/02/02

Research has shown that severe stunting in Tibetan children due to malnutrition is prevalent throughout Tibet, and that morbidity (the prevalence of disease) among Tibetan children is high. A survey by the Tibet Child Nutrition and Collaborative Health Project[24] published in the New England Journal of Medicine in February 2001 found that the overall prevalence of moderate or severe stunting of growth in Tibetan children who were seven years or younger was 51%. This prevalence is classified as very high compared to that of other populations, and is well above that for China as a whole (17%).[25] According to the report, stunting was associated with clinical conditions such as rickets, abdominal distension, hair de-pigmentation, and skin lesions and with a maternal history of hepatitis or goitre. Dr. Nancy Harris and her colleagues,[26] who carried out the research, found that clinical signs of rickets were detected in 66% of the children in the survey area, most of whom were in non-urban areas, and goitre was found in 3% of the children. The study, during August to December of 1994 and 1995, involved the examination of 2,078 Tibetan children from birth to 7 years of age, who were from 11 counties in 5 of the 7 prefectures in the TAR. The 11 counties, which contained more than 50 townships, were representative of the wide range of regions, from urban to nomadic, in Tibet.

23 "Macroeconomics and Health: Investing in Health for Economic Development", cited above
24 The survey was also under the Department of Nutritional Sciences, University of California at Berkeley, the Department of Paediatrics and Medical Research and the Tibet Medical Research Institute, First People's Hospital, Lhasa, TAR. A further report on malnutrition among Tibetan children, "Effects of age, community location, and illness on nutritional status of high altitude Tibetan children, 0-7 years" by Nancy S. Harris, Yeshe Yangzom, Lobsang Pinzo, Palden Gyaltsen, and Patricia B. Crawford, International Paediatric Journal, 1993, can be downloaded from www.ipa-france.net/pubs/inches/inch7_4/hrrs.htm
25 New England Journal of Medicine, 1 February 2001
26 Patricia B Crawford, Yeshe Yangzom, Lobsang Pinzo, Palden Gyaltsen and Mark Hudes.

Moderate and severe stunting among Tibetan children was also documented in 1986 by a UNICEF/TAR Ministry of Child Health survey of 14,272 Tibetan children under seven in Lhasa, and by a Tibet Child Nutrition Project (TCNP) which surveyed 342 children between 1993 and 1995. The urban and rural rates of stunting in the areas under survey were more than twice the levels documented in seven Chinese provinces.[27] A health and nutrition survey, carried out by a western NGO in three counties in the Lhasa Valley during November and December 2001, found that counties further from Lhasa had a considerably higher stunting rate than those close to the capital.[28]

Dr. Harris and her colleagues found evidence that *"stunting of growth as a consequence of chronic malnutrition is often associated with irreversible neuro-developmental delay and increased morbidity and mortality."* Both stunting and failure to gain weight within the normal range are indicators of chronic malnutrition caused by a long-term food deficit or a long-term micronutrient deficit – either the child is not receiving enough food or it is not receiving enough of the right kinds of food.

Various significant micronutrient deficiencies have been documented in Tibetan areas. For example, the TCNP survey referred to above found very low vitamin D levels and significant iron deficiencies. A survey carried out in the Lhasa valley area by a western NGO in the early 1990s found a very high incidence of anaemia among Tibetan 6-12 month old infants – twice as high as the incidence in Chinese children.[29] Scurvy outbreaks (scurvy is a condition characterised by general weakness, anaemia, gum disease and skin haemorrhages resulting from a lack of vitamin C in the diet) still occur in various regions of the TAR. Low selenium and iodine have been documented during studies of Kashin-Beck ('Big Bone') disease.[30] (See Chapter Six)

Other factors that can lead to stunting of growth in children are exposure to infection, other disease and emotional stress. Although the physiological effects of high altitude could also be included as a possible factor, Dr Nancy Harris states in her paper that in this case no association was found between altitude and stunting, indicating that the effect of altitude is not the determining factor in the growth failure of the Tibetan children studied.

27 See: "Effect of economic reforms on child growth in urban and rural areas of China." Shen, T., Habicht, Jp., Chang, Y. NEJM 1996, 335: pps.400-406

28 Report by a western NGO, Tibet Autonomous Region, December 2001

29 Report of a western NGO together with the Lhasa Health Bureau

30 Moreno-Reyes, R., Suetens, C., Mathieu, F., Begaux, F. et al. Kashin-Beck osteoarthropathy in rural Tibet in relation to selenium and iodine status. NEJM 1998; 339 (16): 1112-1120

Dr Harris' research refers to the adverse consequences in later life of childhood stunting – including impaired development, lower intelligence, poorer academic performance, and a reduced capacity for work in adults. An editorial by Glen E Maberly and Kevin M Sullivan, also in the 1 February 2001 edition of New England Journal of Medicine, pointed to the evidence presented by Harris of micronutrient deficiencies *"that constitute a double insult to the developing brains and bodies of Tibetan children, further limiting their ability to reach their genetic potential."*

Dr Harris concludes:

> *"Generalisations about the growth of children living at high altitudes may deflect attention from the urgent need for maternal and child health programmes in Tibet. Malnutrition and common childhood illnesses can be modified by changes in health education and health care. Culturally-specific programmes should be implemented to address the constellation of physiological, socio-economic, agricultural, and environmental factors that affect the health of the children on the Tibetan plateau."*

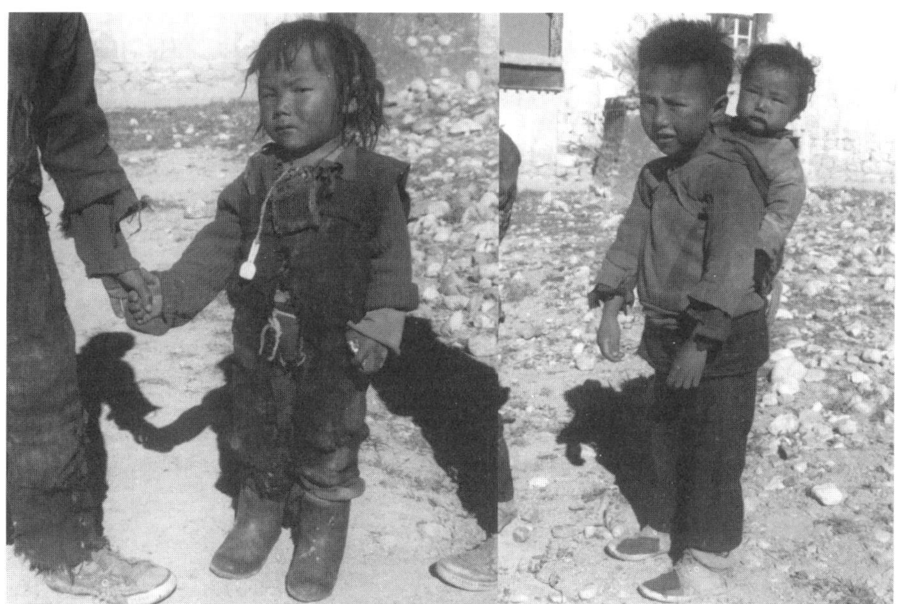

LEFT AND RIGHT young girl and boy in rural Tibet ©Sue Gray/TIN

Tuberculosis

In Tibet, an estimated 5-20% of the population has tuberculosis (TB), which is primarily a disease of the respiratory system, and is spread by coughing and sneezing.[31] TB – which is on the increase worldwide – is a condition commonly associated with poor communities. Multi-drug resistant TB (MDR TB) – a severe form of the condition – also affects people in Tibet, and treatment for this form of TB is too expensive for most Tibetans to afford.[32] China has a national programme to combat tuberculosis,[33] but reports received by TIN suggest that this has so far had a negligible impact in Tibet.[34] TB has an adverse impact on social development, mainly because it tends to affect people between the ages of 20 and 45 who are at the most productive time of their lives, in terms of supporting their families, and contributing to social and economic development. TB patients, if not properly treated, can spread the disease to others; medical studies have found that an active TB patient can spread the condition to about 20 healthy people each year in the first 2 years of the disease.

Dr Mary Maish, who carried out a study on pulmonary disease in Tibet,[35] gives the following reasons why TB remains a problem in Tibet:

> *"First, there is neither a screening programme in place, nor is there any consistency in how patients are identified, treated and followed-up. Also there is a deficiency in patient education with regard to TB that leads to problems of non-compliance. Finally, the movement of people in and out of Tibet as well as within the region itself, has vastly increased in the last 50 years. With the recent influx of Han Chinese, Muslims, Mongolians, Turks and tourists, the amount of TB brought in from other areas has increased and has made the disease more difficult to control."*

31 According to the WHO, which declared TB to be a global emergency in 1993, TB kills approximately 2 million people each year worldwide. The breakdown in health services, the spread of HIV/AIDS and the emergence of multidrug-resistant TB are contributing to the worsening impact of this disease. The WHO estimates that between 2002 and 2020, approximately 1 billion people will be newly infected, over 150 million people will get sick, and 36 million will die of TB if control is not further strengthened. In Eastern Europe and Africa, TB deaths are increasing after almost 40 years of decline. In terms of numbers of cases, the biggest burden of TB is in south-east Asia. According to a report in People's Daily on 23 March 1996, TB kills twice as many Chinese as all the other contagious diseases, and Chinese TB patients, which numbered 6 million in 1996, represent a quarter of the world's total, as quoted in China News Analysis no 1562, 15 June 1996, "Health and Medical Insurance"

32 People with MDR TB disease, a form of TB that is resistant to two or more of the primary drugs used to treat TB, must be treated with special drugs. These drugs are not as effective as the usual drugs for TB and they may cause more side effects. Also, some people with MDR TB disease must see a TB expert who can closely observe their treatment to make sure it is working. People who have spent time with someone sick with MDR TB disease can become infected with TB bacteria that are resistant to several drugs. For a fact sheet on MDR TB see the American Lung Association website at: www.lungusa.org/diseases/mdrtbfac.html

33, 34 & 35 See footnotes on next page

Medical treatment for the condition varies from county to county in both the TAR and Tibetan areas outside the TAR. The Tibet Tuberculosis Control Centre comes under the regional government's Anti-Epidemic Station. In Shigatse (Chi: Rigaze) prefecture, three counties are taking part in pilot projects for Directly Observed Treatment (DOT), where the health worker watches the patient take the medicine every other day. In Meldrogongkar (Chi: Mozhugongka) county in Lhasa Municipality, the county hospital has been admitting TB patients to perform DOT, but this has proved to be impractical and expensive; most places dispense the TB drugs and refill the bottles when the patient returns and shows the empty bottles to the health worker. The township health workers are trained in treating TB at the county level in these three counties – but in the other 15 counties of Shigatse prefecture there are no TB trained staff and patients have to go to the prefectural capital, Shigatse, for treatment. According to one Western NGO, out-of-pocket expenses for treatment can be too high for some Tibetans to afford.[36]

While working in the TAR, one health professional encountered patients suffering from MDR TB, which represents *"a very dangerous situation for the community"*. People with MDR TB disease must be treated with special drugs, which are very expensive, and the condition needs to be monitored closely by medical professionals.[37]

33 (see previous page) According to China's Ten-Year Plan for TB control (1991-2000), state authorities plan to take steps for strengthening work related to TB prevention and treatment. The WHO acknowledged China's initial success in attempting to bring the disease under control at the Fourth World Congress on TB in Washington DC in 2002. The WHO reported that China had managed to bring programmes backed by the WHO to half its population, according to a report in the New Scientist on 3 June 2002

34 (see previous page) A team from the NGO Kham Aid gave the following account of the prevalence of TB during visits to hospitals and clinics in Kardze (Chi: Ganzi) Tibetan Autonomous Prefecture (TAP), Sichuan province (extract from the Kham Aid website, www.khamaid.org): *"On the road coming up to Dartsedo (Chi: Kangding), at a construction site, Bruce [Dr. Bruce Beattie of the charity International SOS, a member of the team] had observed a worker with characteristic signs of TB lymph nodes draining from his neck. The disease is problematic throughout poor rural areas. It is diagnosed by means of a chest X-ray and a skin test. The Dawu (Chi: Daofu county) hospital sees 50-60 cases a year. China has a national program to combat TB, but the doctors in Dawu said that this is having only a small effect. One major hindrance is it's hard to diagnose the afflicted people unless they voluntarily go in for testing. Since many Tibetans don't go in – either because they live too far away, or they are too poor, or too stoic – there are many, many unreported cases"*

35 (see previous page) "Health Care in Tibet: Clinical and Policy Perspectives", Mary Maish MD, Harvard Health Policy Review Spring 2001 Vol. 2 No. 1

36 The same NGO quoted a figure of 400 yuan (US$48) required as a deposit for treatment, presumably where the patient was not covered by the Cooperative Medical Service (CMS). Although this deposit was refundable once the course of treatment was completed, many patients could not afford the initial outlay

37 Prisoners in Tibet are particularly vulnerable to contracting TB and MDR TB. The same health worker told TIN: *"Political prisoners, for instance, are frequently denied medical care until their condition becomes particularly severe and treatment, which is often incomplete, is given. The prisoner is then often released into the community with a multi-drug-resistant TB, which will eventually lead to death and may also be transmitted to their family"*

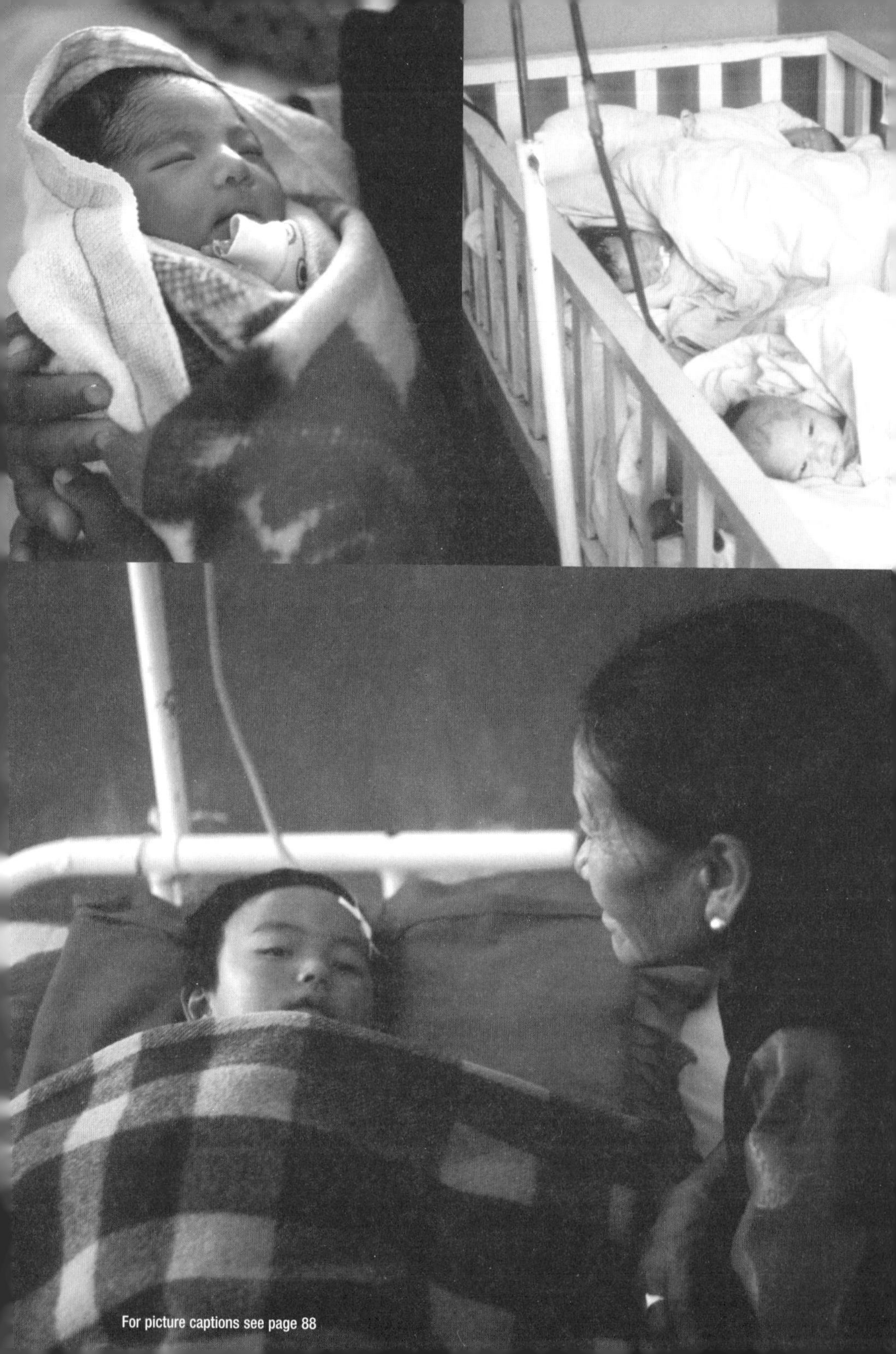

For picture captions see page 88

Chapter Five

Mother and child health

Tibetan women and girls bear a disproportionate part of the burden of poverty, despite the fact that they make up nearly 50% of the general work force and work long hours undertaking work outside the home in addition to childcare and household responsibilities.[1] For Tibetan women of all ages, lack of access to the most basic services remains widespread throughout most of the Tibet Autonomous Region (TAR): the least access to basic education and health care means that pregnancy and childbirth all too often put their health and survival at risk.

Tibetan women living in remote rural areas, far from clinics or hospitals and unable to afford medical treatment, are at particular risk during pregnancy and childbirth. Tibet has a very high maternal mortality rate (MMR), which is at least partially a result of the lack of access to health services for a high proportion of women in rural areas. According to reports from non-governmental organisations (NGOs) with experience of work in Tibet, nearly 90% of women in rural Shigatse (Chi: Rigaze), for instance, deliver their baby at home, with no trained health worker to assist them. The most common causes of maternal death, in order of frequency, are post-partum haemorrhage (haemorrhaging after delivery), eclampsia (toxemia of pregnancy), co-existing medical conditions, obstructed labour and post-partum sepsis (uterine infection). Many women in rural households in the same prefecture did not know about emergencies and danger signs in pregnancy and labour, nor when to call the health worker, even if there is one in the area. International research on childbirth has shown that the most effective intervention that helps reduce death and sickness related to pregnancy is to have a trained health worker, who is capable of treating a post-partum haemorrhage or other complications, present at the delivery.

According to one NGO working in the TAR the barriers to Tibetan women benefiting from care during pregnancy and labour include the following:[2]

- Lack of knowledge
- Distance to clinic
- Lack of transport
- Lack of money

1 A Western donor to health projects in Tibet concluded the following after involvement in social research: *"Women represent 46% of the labour force in the TAR and perform some 70% of the farm work. They also take primary responsibility for managing household resources, such as water and fuel, and play the main role in ensuring food security, education and socialisation and family health care. However, they rarely participate in community affairs or decision-making in the rural areas and few women fill management or technical positions in the city"*

2 The same obstacles are likely to apply in Tibetan areas outside the TAR

- No faith in the health system
- Traditional beliefs surrounding birth
- Poor skills of medical personnel at township level
- Staff attitude to people from villages
- Run-down and unhygienic clinic buildings
- Medical staff are male not female

The same NGO found that from a sample survey of village women in the TAR, only 6% of women who gave birth in a 12-month period were attended by someone trained in clean and safe deliveries. Responses from the villagers to various questions in the survey about difficulties in child-birth included the following:

> *"We want to have babies in the hospital but transportation is very difficult. It is also very expensive to have a baby in the hospital, so we give birth in the home and wait for the gods' decision on how it will turn out (death or life). ...The women would like to go to the hospital to have prenatal care, but they have little or no money. Also, there are problems with road access, and the transportation itself (like tractors) is not appropriate. The women also do not receive enough information regarding what methods are available to prevent pregnancy. ...One of the reasons why we don't call a doctor is a custom in this village, the other reason is that the women are too shy to call the doctor. But when we see the serious signs* [of prolonged labour, lasting four to five days], *we usually call upon a doctor, if the doctor cannot do anything, he will suggest that we bring the patient to the township or county hospital and the village doctor will follow us. ...The foremost problem is transportation and women are worried that children will be delivered on the way to the hospital, especially in the summertime as most roads are washed away by floods and cannot be crossed."*

Due to their high level of responsibility and workload, Tibetan mothers are often forced to return to work as soon as one month after delivering a child, and hence exclusive breast-feeding is very rarely practised. The working mother will feed the baby in the morning and may return from the fields to feed again at lunchtime. The baby will then be fed again when the mother returns home at night. During the day the child is given a mixture of other foods and drinks, often by the grandparents. *Tsampa* porridge is often introduced within a few weeks of birth and *dri* (female yak) or cow's milk. There is a greatly increased risk of diarrhoea due to lack of hygiene in preparing the milk and other foods for the child, which can result in malnutrition for the child. The early introduction of inappropriate foods along with inadequate breast-feeding can result in basic nutritional deficiencies from an early age. (See Chapters Three and Four)

Divinations and disease

A female health consultant who has worked in the TAR gave the following account of a meeting convened among Tibetan women and western NGO consultants in 2001.

> *"The major illnesses experienced by the women were bad colds, flu, lung infections, appendicitis, and diarrhoea. The women were asked to talk about what were the greatest difficulties in their lives. One mentioned looking after the animals, milking, feeding them and fetching water with a bucket on a stick – while at the same time caring for small children. Her husband, however, did the herding in the day-time. Most of the women agreed with her. Asked what they do if their children are sick, several said they first checked with the lamas and were usually advised to take their children to hospital, which they then did. However, if the child was near death, they would have divinations done*[3] *and prayers said. The choice of hospital was dependent on wealth. There were no facilities for operations or in-patients at the local clinic. In the event of illness Western medicine was chosen for immediate effect, while Tibetan traditional medicine was the treatment of choice for long-term ailments."*

Infant and maternal mortality

The Chinese authorities claimed that maternal and infant mortality rates had dropped to a 'historic low' in 2002, and linked this decrease to the 'democratic reforms' in Tibet since 1959. Zhang Wengkang, Minster of Health, stated in May (2002) that maternal death in child-birth had dropped from 715.8 per 10,000 to 324.7 per 10,000 in 2001.[4] The same report stated that infant mortality[5] had dropped from 91.8 per 1,000 to 31.3 per 1,000 in 2001.[6] The reliability of these statistics is not known; Chinese birth and infant mortality calculations are known to be under-reported.[7]

3 The reference to 'divination' is likely to refer to the performance of a ritual to propitiate protective deities

4 Report on a speech given on 29 May 2002 by Zhang Wenkang to the 3rd National Health Aid to Tibet Work Forum. The report was entitled: "Serve the overall situation, continue to exert ourselves: work hard to carry out well Health Aid to Tibet work at the start of the new century", published in Health and Government Administration News (Vol 9) and republished on the Chinese Ministry of Health website

5 The death of infants under 1 year old

6 For a chart on comparative infant mortality rates worldwide see: www.bartleby.com/151/a28.html The same survey, from The World Factbook 2001 states that the highest figure of infant mortality is for Angola, at 193.72 deaths per 1,000 live births. The figures for Afghanistan are also high, at 147.02 deaths per 1,000 live births. The infant mortality rate for the UK is 5.54 deaths per 1,000 live births and the figure for the US is 6.76 deaths per 1,000 births

7 Researcher Giovanni Merli, who attempted to test the reliability of such data in Zibo City in Shandong province, wrote: *"In the evaluation of the quality of Chinese demographic data, both western and Chinese scholars agree that Chinese birth and infant mortality systems suffer from severe under-reporting, and that censuses, surveys and registration systems are complicated by respondents failing to report births and infant deaths".* China Quarterly, No 155, September 1998, quoted in Jasper Becker, "The Chinese" (John Murray 2000)

A study conducted in 16 Tibetan counties by the Chinese National Ministry of Public Health in 1989 stated that the mortality rate among infants (under one year old) was 92 per 1000 in the Tibetan counties, as compared with 68 per 1000 in the rest of China; the mortality rate among children less than 5 years old was 127 per 1,000, as compared with 84 per 1,000, and the maternal mortality rate was 73 per 10,000 as compared with 20 per 10,000.[8] According to the study, pneumonia was responsible for 41% and diarrhoea for 20% of deaths in infants in the TAR.[9] These conclusions backed up the findings of a separate survey by Dr Nancy Harris published in the New England Journal of Medicine on 1 February 2001 (See Chapter Four, Poverty and Health).[10]

An analysis of Chinese government census statistics for the year 1990, by researcher Fergus Thomas,[11] found that rather than declining, childhood mortality rates had in fact increased in the period before the census. Thomas concluded that *"using Tibet's childhood mortality as a proxy for development would rank the region as one of the least developed places on earth."*[12]

It has been acknowledged by experts on socio-economic development that one of the most powerful contributors to reduced child mortality is the literacy of mothers, which is the result of an education system that ensures widespread access to education for the poor, including girls as well as boys. According to World Bank estimates, for each year of education for girls, child mortality is cut by 10%, female fertility is reduced by 10% and wages are boosted by 10 to 20%. In poor rural areas of Tibet, families often require the children for productive labour. In the TAR, if children have the opportunity to study it is often the girls who will be withdrawn from the education system first. Often Tibetan families can simply not afford to send their children to school, due to fees imposed for education in Tibetan areas.[13]

8 National Centre of Health Information and Statistics, MCH baseline study, People's Republic of China: National Ministry of Public Health, 1989, cited in "Nutritional and Health Status of Tibetan children living at high altitudes", by Dr Nancy Harris MD et al, New England Journal of Medicine, Vol 344, No 5, 1 February 2001, pps 341-7

9 Ministry of Public Health Information and Statistics National Centre of Health Statistics, China 1989

10 Various statistics on infant and child mortality have been given at different periods by the Chinese authorities and by NGOs operating in Tibetan areas. A further figure on infant mortality was given in a report by the Chinese Ministry of Foreign Affairs of the People's Republic of China in 2000. The Ministry stated that the infant mortality rate dropped from 91.8 per thousand in 1989 to 61.96 per thousand in 1992 in 20 counties of the TAR. A 1995 study by G Dankert and Zhang Weiguo "Indirect methods to determine mortality: Tibetans in the People's Republic of China": Teaching text of the Institute of Social Studies, Population and Development, The Hague, gave a high estimate of infant mortality in the TAR based on analysis of mortality and sex differentials of the Tibetan population of the TAR (quoted in: "Fertility and its control in the Tibet Autonomous Region: an Analysis of the Fertility Data in the 1990 Census of the Xizang Autonomous Region", by Fergus Thomas, a report submitted in partial fulfilment of the requirement of the MSc degree in Medical Demography, London School of Hygiene and Tropical Medicine, University of London, August 2000). Dankert and Zhang applied the Brass technique for estimating childhood mortality, estimating a male Infant Mortality Rate (IMR) of 170 per thousand and a male Childhood Mortality Rate (CMR) of 52 per thousand for males. For females the rates are calculated at IMR: 128 per thousand and CMR at 38 per thousand. This data for childhood mortality places Tibet alongside some of the world's least developed nations

11 "Fertility and its control in the Tibet Autonomous Region: an Analysis of the Fertility Data in the 1990 Census of the Xizang Autonomous Region", a report submitted in partial fulfilment of the requirement of the MSc degree in Medical Demography, London School of Hygiene and Tropical Medicine, University of London, August 2000)

12 & 13 See footnotes on next page

The incidence and treatment of sexually transmitted infections

Staff in prefecture hospitals say that they have seen a steady increase in the number of sexually transmitted infections (STIs) in Tibetan areas in recent years. Statistical data on STIs in Tibetan areas is not available, but the available accounts of an increase in Tibet may reflect the increase in commercial sex workers in urban areas. The large number of recently opened private clinics in Lhasa that advertise 'cures' for STIs supports this view (see the section on HIV/AIDS in Chapter Six).

Most health workers, particularly at the township level, do not have the skills to diagnose STIs nor do they have access to any laboratory testing. Even when an STI is correctly diagnosed, treatment is often inappropriate. The most common treatment for any type of vaginal discharge is douching (an ineffective treatment for STIs), and if the symptoms continue, intravenous antibiotics, which are expensive and usually incorrectly administered. Gonorrhoea is reportedly the most common sexually transmitted infection, although other STIs may be under-diagnosed. The blood test for syphilis is available at most hospitals that have a laboratory but there are currently no testing facilities for chlamydia in the TAR – one of the most common STIs in most parts of the world.

According to one NGO, a survey of more than a thousand women in various townships in the TAR found that 65% of the surveyed group had reproductive health problems ranging from minor gynaecological problems to STIs. The risk of infection for rural women is thought to be increasing, as the men of the household now travel long distances to urban areas in order to seek employment, and may during these absences use the services of commercial sex workers. The concept of using condoms to prevent STIs is not widely recognised or well understood by most people and in urban areas where condoms are available, expense limits their use.

12 (see previous page) Fergus Thomas, ibid

13 (see previous page) The then TAR government chairman, Gyaltsen Norbu, announced at the end of 1993 that one third of children in the TAR were unable to afford to go to school (reported by Xinhua, 5 June 1994). For further background on funding and access to education see "Education in Tibet: Policy and Practice since 1950" by Catriona Bass, TIN/Zed Books, 1998

Reproductive health

When asked about reproductive health issues, women in Tibet express their desire for access to cheap and safe contraception so that they can control their own fertility. However, township and village health workers do not discuss reproductive goals with women prior to dispensing contraceptives and they do not generally have the skills to screen women and choose which form of contraceptive is the most appropriate. The availability, cost and type of contraceptives varies greatly between counties and frequently there is no choice to be made due to the availability of only one method of contraceptive. Methods of contraception are generally targeted at women; it is rare for men to be sterilised. Condoms are available only in urban areas and rural families have little knowledge of them.

Interviews by one NGO with township level health workers in two counties in the TAR found that health workers did not know how to manage common complications related to contraceptive use. Complaints of back pain and excessive menstrual bleeding commonly associated with intra-uterine devices (IUDs) were not understood. One township doctor who was interviewed[14] said: "*When* [the patient] *complained of pain and discomfort* [after insertion of an IUD] *I told her to switch to the oral contraceptives*". Another health worker said "*I've seen a few women who complain of vaginal bleeding after taking oral contraceptives, I tell them to stop the medicine and give them an anti-bleeding injection*" (irregular vaginal bleeding is a common, usually benign side-effect during the first few months of oral contraceptive use).

Another survey found that 23% of women complained of side-effects from contraceptive use, the most common of these complaints being back pain, kidney problems, headaches and bleeding. Women reported the following factors as barriers to the use of contraceptives: lack of availability; high costs; the need to travel a long distance to the township clinic or county hospital that provides family planning; a lack of knowledge and information regarding the different family planning options available; being so weak after birth (anaemia and/or malnutrition) that hospitals refuse to give contraceptives (this refers to sterilisation and IUD insertion); and illiteracy, which can result in the contraceptive pill being taken improperly.

The availability and cost of contraceptives varies widely and most township clinics have a very limited choice of contraceptives provided to them by the county hospital. Stock is frequently found to be beyond its expiry date, and few township doctors are actually trained to insert an IUD or a hormonal implant under the skin of the arm.

14 A report from a Western NGO

Although in some areas contraceptive pills are distributed to them to dispense free of charge, the majority of village doctors do not provide contraception. For surgical sterilisation (tubal ligation), it would generally be necessary for a women to travel to the county or prefectural hospital. However, lack of transport and money frequently prevent women from travelling to the main towns where these services are available.

The county health bureau is responsible for sending mobile teams to the townships to provide contraception free of charge. They may provide the Norplant hormonal implant,[15] the IUD and/or sterilisation. It is the job of the local women's association to identify married women who already have the quota of children officially allowed and who are not taking contraception to ensure that they are aware that the mobile family planning team is coming to their township. Reports indicate that woman who already have 2 or 3 children are sometimes put under strong pressure to go to these mobile clinics. The implementation of this system varies greatly between counties and between prefectures, and many rural women say that these teams never come to their area.

These differences in the availability of family planning methods in Tibetan areas have been highlighted in a number of surveys undertaken by Western health workers. One survey of family planning methods, conducted in 7 rural villages in the TAR, interviewed over 500 households and found that 40% of married women reported using some form of family planning; 78% had an IUD, 17% used condoms, 2% oral contraceptives, 2% injectable birth-control hormone (Depo Provera)[16] and 1% had opted for sterilisation.

A survey in counties that were rural but located within the Lhasa Municipality found over 50% of mothers used contraception – 34% of these women were using oral contraceptives, 17% IUDs, 12% injectable birth-control hormone, 9% hormonal implants, and 28% had been sterilised. A further survey, of rural women in two counties in the TAR, found that only 20% of married women in the areas under study were using a method of contraception. 10% used oral contraceptives, 5% used an IUD, 3% injectable birth control hormone and 0.4% surgical abortion.

The prices of contraceptives also vary by location – in some areas free contraceptives are available, and in others areas women have to pay up to 100 yuan (US$12) for an intra-uterine device and 200 yuan (US$24) for surgical sterilisation. Women living in urban areas of Tibet have better access to family planning and therefore more choices are available to them. The number of women in urban areas requesting surgical abortion has been reported by some prefectural level hospitals to represent nearly 30% of all visits to the out-patient department.

15 The implants are six matchstick size rods inserted into the upper arm. Norplant implants give off very small amounts of a hormone much like the progesterone a woman produces during the last two weeks of each monthly cycle

16 Like the Pill and Norplant, Depo-Provera contains a hormone similar to progesterone. It is given by injection, generally 4 times a year

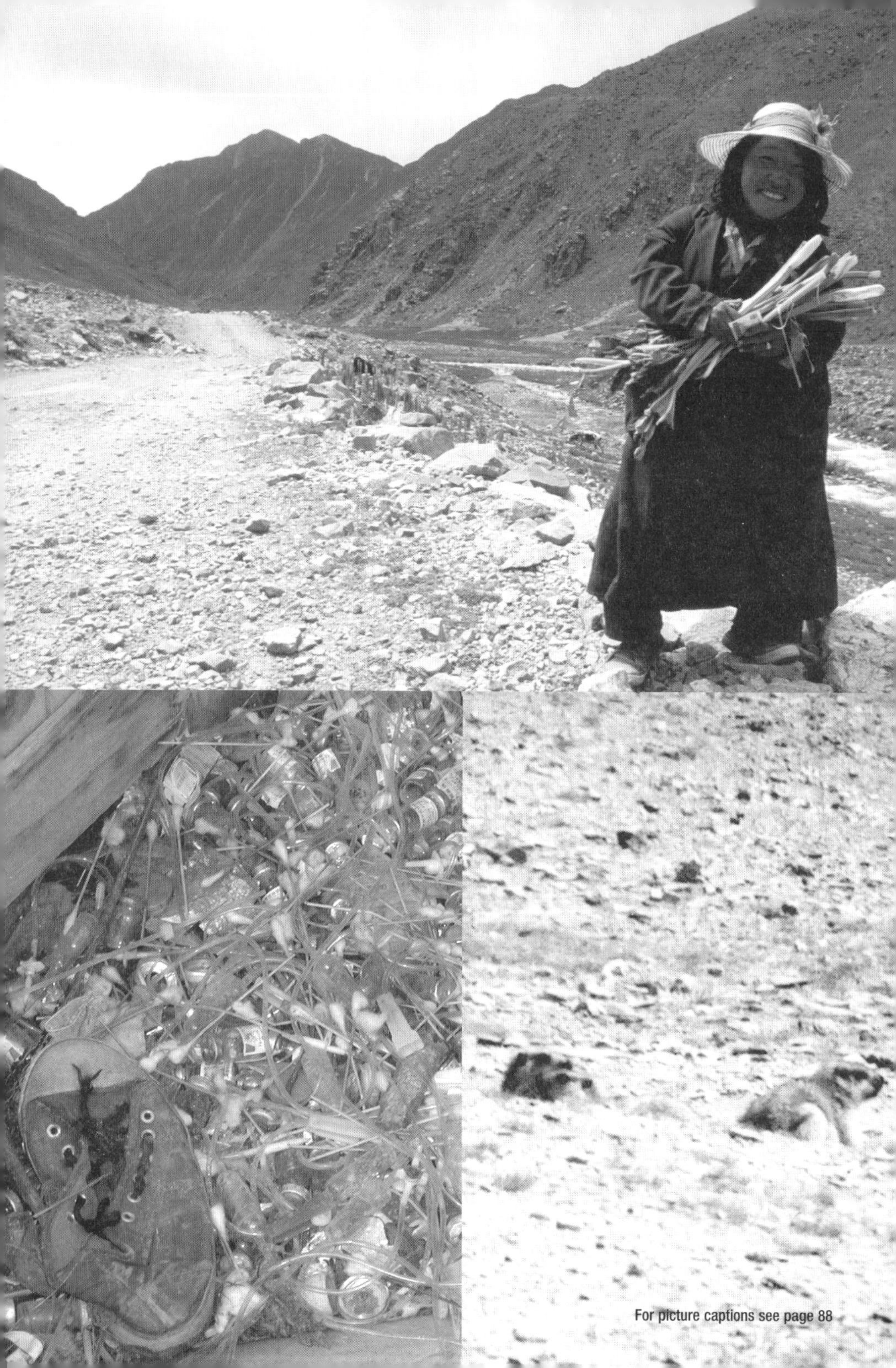

For picture captions see page 88

Chapter Six

Strategies and prevention

Iodine Deficiency Disorders (IDD) – known as 'the hidden hunger' – cause widespread physical and psychological ill-health in Tibet, but can normally be addressed by supplementation of iodine. The research presented below explains the measures taken by the authorities to deal with this condition and the impact at grass-roots level. This chapter also assesses the effectiveness, or otherwise, of strategies to deal with other fundamental health concerns in Tibet – outbreaks of the plague, which still occur in some Tibetan areas, and Kashin-Beck or 'Big Bone' disease, which deforms, and in the worst cases incapacitates, significant numbers of farmers and herders in rural areas. There is also a need to address the impact of more 'modern' diseases. The section on HIV/AIDS shows how the possibility of an epidemic in Tibetan areas is now being taken seriously by the authorities, but that the difficulties and delays in the development of preventive strategies could prove extremely damaging in the long-term.

The treatment of Iodine Deficiency Disorders (IDD)

The World Health Organisation (WHO) estimates that IDD affects over 740 million people – 13% of the world's population – and 30% of the remainder are at risk. IDD poses serious public health problems in 130 developing countries; nearly 50 million people suffer from some degree of IDD-related brain damage.[1] Iodine is an essential micro-nutrient required in both animals and humans for the synthesis of thyroid hormones which regulate normal growth and development of the brain and nervous system, and are essential for maintenance of body heat and energy. IDD can result in still-births, brain damage leading to cretinism in the foetus, loss of energy due to thyroid deficiency and retarded physical development. IDD also causes goitre, which brings other complications such as hypothyroidism, which slows down the metabolism of the body. Cretinism, which is the result of foetal iodine deficiency, is expressed in stunted physical growth and mental retardation. The term cretinism describes two different conditions. The first includes severe hypothyroidism, dry swollen skin and tongue, deep hoarse voice, apathy and mental deficiency. In the second condition, which is a neurological type of cretinism, the person exhibits mental defects, deaf mutism, paralysis and a spastic rigidity that usually affects the legs.

1 See the WHO website at: www.who.int/nut/idd.htm

However, according to a report by Hanne Klink Jensen,[2] who has worked in Tibet for Medecins Sans Frontieres (MSF), the most devastating effects of IDD on a population are the results of milder IDD, including more subtle mental impairment and reduced physical aptitude among children and adults: *"This mental impairment during the learning period and the lethargy and lack of initiative in the adults suffering from IDD can have great consequences for the development of a community. If IDD is widespread, these manifestations can have social and economic effects on the country as a whole."*

IDD can be eliminated only through iodine supplementation in the deficient communities. Salt iodisation is the main long-term supplementation method, with iodine capsules and injections as intermediate measures.[3] The authorities in Tibet are currently taking action to reduce the incidence of IDD in certain areas. According to Klink Jensen's report, the distribution of iodised salt by the authorities is working well in large, urban areas, including Lhasa, where most of the affected population are now consuming authorised iodised salt. However, coverage and uptake in rural villages remains very low. A Tibetan doctor who worked in rural areas near Lhasa confirmed that there had been improvement in people's health following the introduction of iodised salt. The doctor told TIN: *"Doctors* [in the area] *participated in a campaign, which included television coverage, to educate the public on the use of iodised salt. We went to the villages to give advice. At first people were not receptive to this advice, they had the attitude that there was nothing that could be done about the problem of goitres."*

In June 1998 the Tibet Autonomous Region (TAR) government passed legislation that enforces the purchase of iodised salt. At the same time a strengthened system was implemented to block the traditional sources of salt from Tibetan nomad traders. For hundreds of years, villagers in central Tibet have traded barley for rock salt brought by the nomads from lakes in Nagchu (Chi: Naqu) prefecture. The nomads who inhabit the area dig out the salt from the lakes and prepare it for transport; in December, when the nomads are ready to take their animals to lower grounds for the last grazing possibilities of the season, the rock salt is loaded onto sheep, yaks or trucks and traded in villages and the market in county towns. One objective within the enforcement programme is to catch and fine the nomads, and confiscate the unauthorised salt. Also, according to Klink Jensen, although the salt that is iodised at the plant in Lhasa comes from the same place where the nomads have dug out salt for centuries, the nomads have not been invited to participate in the work.

2 "Mountains of Salt: An analysis of the Iodine Deficiency Disorders" by Hanne Klink Jensen: Degree Project report series, 1999:3, Master of Science Programme in International Health 20-Point Project Work, Uppsala University, Uppsala, Sweden, June 1999. TIN is grateful to the author for permission to base this section on information from the report

3 The International Council for the Control of Iodine Deficiency Disorders. On 18 March 1991 the then Chinese Premier Li Peng pledged that China would eliminate IDD by the year 2000, according to China News Analysis, No 1562, 15 June 1996. In September 1993 the State Council passed a General Plan to this effect and on 6 January 1994 a Directive strengthened the management of the table salt market and barred non-iodized salt from iodine-deficient regions

Klink Jensen gives an example of the enforcement of the scheme in her report following interviews with villages in a county in the TAR.[4] The villagers told the IDD researchers that in December 1998, following the passing of legislation on iodised salt, the authorities told them that they must buy salt from the government and that trading of salt with the nomads was prohibited.

Klink Jensen writes:

> *"The villagers were unhappy and sad about the decision. Several people expressed their concern that with no salt trade the nomads would not come back to their villages. Serious concern was expressed about the well-being of the nomads. Villagers said that the nomads would be in a very bad and difficult situation if they cannot trade salt and get their supply of barley and wheat to take back to the high plateau for the winter. Everybody knew that the nomads had an extremely hard winter* [the year before] *due to excessive snowstorms. Many nomads had lost large numbers of animals and were still suffering from the loss. The villagers said that they would have to buy the salt from the authorities. When asked if they could refuse, they laughed and said that they really had no choice. If they refused they would be punished one way or another. Not many of the villagers had tried the salt from the authorities before, but two women in the village said: "The salt is no good, it is kind of sweet tasting and to make butter tea you must add much more of the government salt than of the rock salt." The village leader "expected that many villagers would have problems in paying cash for the salt because of the bad economic situation."*

4 The name of the village has been withheld

5 (see next page) An alternative to taking in iodine through salt is to add iodine to local water supplies. This method is documented in the following reports: "Control of iodine deficiency using iodination of water in a goitre endemic area", Elnagar, Babikir; Elton, Mohammed; and Karlsson, F. Anders, International Journal of Food Sciences and Nutrition, Basingstoke, March 1997 and "Dynamics of Environmental Supplementation of Iodine: Four Years' Experience of Iodination of Irrigation Water in Hotien, Xinjiang, China", Xin-Min, Jiang et al, Archives of Environmental Health, Vol 52 (6), November/December 1997

6 (see next page) Klink Jensen quotes WHO research in 1994: "Indications for Assessing Iodine Deficiency Disorders and their Control through Salt Iodisation". The possible side effects of excess intake of dietary iodine are the development of iodide goitre, thyrotoxicosis due to elevated levels of thyroid hormones creating a rapid heart rate, excessive sweating, instability and loss of weight. Hashimotos thyroiditis, iodide and colloid goitre, and thyroid carcinoma can also be seen in rare cases. People over 40 years of age with life-long iodine deficiency are especially at risk

Hanne Klink Jensen's report concludes that while the iodine supplementation plan in Tibet is well in keeping with international guidelines (salt is being iodised, and penalties are being put into effect),[5] a closer look at how the plan is implemented reveals major difficulties within the system. The first difficulty is that the level of iodisation of salt is set according to international standards, which assume that the average person on a daily basis consumes 5-15 grams of salt per day. However, due to the special diet of the Tibetans, the fact that their main fluid intake comes from butter tea, and because a higher intake of fluid is needed at high altitudes, Tibetans have a much higher intake of salt than the international average. This has not been taken into account in determining how much iodine should be added to salt in Tibet – as a result the Tibetans who use iodised salt may be taking in very large amounts of iodine, which may cause disease in susceptible individuals.[6] Klink Jensen suggests that research should be carried out on the dietary habits of Tibetans and their daily consumption of salt as part of the IDD programme.

She also recommends the consideration of a subsidy system, as the production price in the TAR, which is the Lhasa price, is heavily increased as transport costs are added to the salt price. Klink Jensen also makes the following comments about IDD and traditional Tibetan medicine:

> *"The official IDD programme makes no attempt to co-operate with the traditional Tibetan medical community. This is a missed opportunity... Many Tibetans would go first to Tibetan doctors for treatment before turning to the government clinics and hospitals... Because Tibetan medicine is based on imbalances in the person, including imbalances in diet, there is already a meeting point between this tradition and western medicine when it comes to the prevention and treatment of IDD. The herbal medicines used in the traditional treatment of goitre may contain iodine, as might the special salt described by the Tibetan doctors. Tibetan doctors may accept iodine capsules and iodised salt if these supplements are explained to them. The support of Tibetan doctors of a supplementation programme would definitely improve its acceptance in the local community."*

According to information in Klink Jensen's report, legislation and enforcement are considered by informed health workers to be premature in the Tibetan IDD programme. Health workers have pointed out that public education in the field of iodine in Tibet is still inadequate and is necessary in order to make the IDD programme sustainable and successful. This advice has not been followed by the central government which has decided to enforce punishments despite the lack of education and knowledge about IDD in the community.

5 & 6 See footnotes on previous page
7 Health Policy Challenges in the TAR: A December 2000 report from US Embassy, Beijing

Kashin-Beck ('Big Bone') disease

Kashin-Beck disease is a debilitating bone disorder that slows bone growth and triggers a gradual stiffening of the major joints. The disease stunts children's growth and inflicts chronic athritis-like pain on adults. According to MSF, the disease is common in a geographical 'crescent' running from the Tibetan plateau across China to Siberia, and there are more than 3 million sufferers among the 30 million people living in the endemic areas. Tibet is one of the most severely affected regions worldwide, with the prevalence rate as high as 80% in some villages in central Tibet, mostly Chamdo (Chi: Changdu) prefecture and Nagchu (Chi: Naqu) prefecture.[7]

As children develop, their soft tissue turns into bone. In adults, a layer of cartilage remains to help ease wear and tear at the joints. Kashin-Beck disease kills the cartilage (elastic tissue), which prevents the bones from growing to their full length and causes the remaining bone cells to accumulate at swelling joints. The disease has a particularly strong impact in farming communities, where livelihoods are threatened as farmers find their ability to work the land curtailed by severe pain and difficulty in grasping farm tools.

Scientists are still attempting to ascertain the exact cause of the disease, and so far three major environmental factors have been isolated as follows: (i) severe cereal contamination by mycotoxin-producing fungi; (ii) selenium and/or iodine deficiency, (iii) high organic matter concentrations in drinking water.[8] Analyses of soil and grain samples in China and Tibet have shown that low selenium concentrations coincide with most, but not all, regions where people are affected by the disease. A Belgian-led team of researchers to Tibet concluded that two-thirds of a sample of 575 children from 12 Tibetan villages had severe iodine deficiency. Half of the children had Kashin-Beck disease, and the team concluded that iodine deficiency is also a contributory factor to Big Bone disease.[9] MSF's research and medical activities in Tibet has focused on this illness, and MSF has carried out preventive work including supplying iodine, selenium and vitamins C and E as well as improving the quality and storage of basic food supplies such as grain. MSF has also tried to ensure access to clean drinking water – in Lhasa, Shigatse (Chi: Rigaze) and Lhokha (Chi: Shannan) prefectures, it developed 164 clean rural drinking sources between 1993 and 1999 – and community education in hygiene. Physiotherapy treatment programmes instituted by MSF, which involve the training of Tibetan health workers in physiotherapy, help to alleviate the pain of Kashin-Beck disease sufferers.

8 Cahiers d'etudes et de recherches francophones/Agricultures. Vol 9, Issue 2, March – April 2000. Authors: Eric Haubruge, Camille Chasseur, Francoise Mathieu, Francoise Begaux, Francois Malaisse, Nicole Nolard, Dong Zhu, Carl Suetens, Charles Gaspar
9 The New England Journal of Medicine, 15 October 1998; the team was led by Dr Rodrigo Moreno-Reyes of the Universite Libre de Bruxelles in Brussels, Belgium

The plague

In recent years the Chinese authorities have admitted to the existence of epidemics of plague in China and Tibet, although at a local level an outbreak of plague can be something of a taboo subject.

One of the first signs of plague is a very painful, usually swollen, and often hot-to-the-touch lymph-node, called a *bubo*. Another symptom is a rosy rash on the skin. The Black Death of the 14th century in Europe is mainly attributed to bubonic plague. These symptoms, accompanied with fever and extreme exhaustion along with a history of possible exposure to rodents, rodent fleas, wild rabbits, or sick or dead carnivores should lead to suspicion of plague. The disease progresses rapidly and the bacteria can invade the bloodstream, producing severe illness, called plague septicaemia.

Once a human is infected, a progressive and potentially fatal illness generally results unless specific antibiotic therapy is given. Progression leads to blood infection, then, finally, to lung infection. The infection of the lung is termed plague pneumonia, and it can be transmitted to others through the expulsion of infective respiratory droplets by coughing, by a person or animal.

The incubation period of primary pneumonic plague is 1-3 days and is characterised by the development of an overwhelming pneumonia with a high fever, cough, bloody sputum, and chills. For plague pneumonia patients, the death rate is over 50%. Plague is transmitted from animal to animal and from animal to human by the bites of infective fleas. Less frequently, the organism enters through a break in the skin by direct contact with tissue or body fluids of a plague-infected animal, for instance, in the process of skinning a rabbit or other animal. Transmission of plague from person to person but can occur as a factor in plague epidemics in some developing countries. As attempts to eliminate wild rodent plague are costly and futile, primary preventive measures worldwide are directed toward reducing the threat of infection in humans in high-risk areas. This is being done through four main techniques: environmental management, public health education, preventive drug therapy, and vaccines.[10] Globally, the WHO reports 1,000 to 3,000 cases of plague every year.[11]

10 For further information on these measures and a map showing world distribution of the plague in 1998 see: www.cdc.gov/ncidod/dvbid/plague/

11 See the website: www.cdc.gov/ncidod/dvbid/plague/ In the United States, the last urban plague epidemic occurred in Los Angeles in 1924-5. Since then, human plague in the US as occurred as mostly scattered cases in rural areas. The last reported cases of plague in Europe occurred after World War II

In November 1994 China's Health Daily issued a report stating that some 202,000 sq. miles (600,000 sq. km) of the country was infected, with 216 cities and counties host to the plague bacteria. Health Daily reported: *"In Yunnan, the plague epidemic situation pushes into the hinterland from the Burmese border. While in Tibet, 26% of the population live in plague epidemic areas."* The article stated that the provinces of Xinjiang and Qinghai have a plague outbreak almost every year, and also stated: *"In the past few years, the plague has attacked some men and animals in epidemic proportions. It could erupt and spread at any time."*[12] An official pamphlet, "Medicare Service in Tibet" by Zhang Yun, published in 1999, states the following: *"Plague hit the TAR in recent years. Health departments at various levels made great efforts in the last two years to cope with the situation, thus effectively checking the spread of plague."*[13] A Western health professional who has worked in the TAR told TIN: *"There are still outbreaks of plague in Tibet today, but it is a taboo subject and the health authorities do not want to talk about it. Once we approached a particular rural area and it was sealed off, we were told that people there had the plague, and we were not allowed to go anywhere near it."*

Chinese scientists reported that 64 episodes of human plague occurred in Qinghai province (which incorporates part of the Tibetan traditional area of Amdo) during the period 1975-1997.[14] Ten of them were caused by infected Tibetan sheep, which the scientists stated were named as the second most common cause of the plague in Qinghai province, and as such played an important role in the epidemiology of the disease. A survey of livestock carried out in an area of Gansu in 1998 by Chinese scientists found that seven strains of the plague virus *yesinia pestis* were isolated from 2.885 animals, and that one episode of human plague occurred.[15]

Birds and marmots, common in Tibet's grasslands, are also sometimes carriers of the plague, although this applies less in the higher altitude areas, where the cold dry climate does not allow fleas to proliferate. A further study in China's Endemic Diseases Bulletin[16] stated that the marmot was the main source of infection causing pneumonic plague in human beings in China; the major route of plague transmission was through rodent contact. The same paper stated that the death rate from 63 cases of human plague occurring between 1959 and 1988 in Gansu province was 60.3%.

12 "Plague Endemic to China, Tibet", UPI Beijing, 2 November 1994

13 Published by China Intercontinental Press, p 18

14 "Epidemiological analysis of human plague caused by infected Tibetan sheep in Qinghai", Wang Zuyun, Luosong Dawei, Wang ZY, Luosong DW, in Endemic Diseases Bulletin 1999, 14:3, 35-36

15 "The plague control and analysis of its epidemic situation in Gansu in 1998", Xi Jinxiao, Shi Yanlong, Liang Xiaocheng, Shi Yingxiang, Xi-JX, Shi YL, Liang XC, Shi YX, Endemic Diseases Bulletin 1999, 14:4, 51-52, 59

16 "A study on the epidemiological characters and control measures of human plague in Gansu province", Zhang Rongguang (et al), 1994, 9: 4, 22-26; 6 ref

17 (see next page) "A study on the epidemic patterns and control measures of human plague in Qinghai province", Zhu Jinqin, Wu Wenlian, Li Yongzhong, Liu Guang, Wang Chengming, Zhu JQ, Wu WL, Li YZ, Wang CM, Endemic Diseases Bulletin, 1993, 8: 1, 1-8

The authors of the study concluded:

> *"The primary cases had always had contact with animals and their frequency of bubonic plague and septicemia was very high. Based on these findings, some practical measures have been implemented and since 1963, human plague in the province has decreased, with no more cases since 1989."*

A study of 166 human *yersinia pestis* epidemics,[17] which occurred between 1958 and 1992 in Qinghai, also found that marmots acted as a major infectious reservoir for up to 73.5% of the epidemics:

> *"Of the 391 human cases, those of bubonic and septicaemic plague were caused predominantly by the skinning and mealing of infected marmots or wild animals and were liable to change to secondary pneumonia, which comprised 47.7% of cases. Pneumonic epidemics spread directly from person to person via the respiratory tract accounted for 47.1%, while infection via rodents to fleas and to people was only 2.3%.*
>
> *Clinical patterns consisted of mainly pneumonic (57.4%), simple bubonic (23.8%) and septicaemic cases (16.3%)... Fatality rates were 53.8% in pneumonic cases, 28.6% in bubonic and even 100% in septicaemic ones. The cure rate was up to 95.3% where effective treatment was instigated. Appropriate steps have been taken in Qinghai which have reduced the apparent incidence rate since 1984."*

A further study from the Endemic Diseases Bulletin published in 1995[18] reported on 11 episodes of human plague in the TAR, occurring mostly in July-August at the time of abundant rainfall and high temperatures, as well as in the main period of activity of the principal reservoir host, the marmot (the other main infection source was sheep). A total of 84 people, mainly herders and farmers, were infected and 50 died. Early cases were confirmed as having had direct contact with infected animals.

17 See footnote on previous page

18 "Study on the epidemiological characteristics of plague in Tibet and its control strategy", Xirao Ruodeng, Ciren Dunzhu, Xirao RD, Ciren DZ, issue 10: 3, 20-26

19 (see next page) A fuller exploration of the issue of HIV/AIDS in Tibet is beyond the scope of this report but will be featured in a forthcoming TIN publication

20 (see next page) A statistic of 1 million was given in China Daily, 11/10/02. Press reports from Beijing state that China detected its first AIDS patient (a foreign tourist) in 1985, and specialists estimated that the number of carriers in China increased to 500,000 by 1998

21 (see next page) David Murphy, the Far Eastern Economic Review correspondent in Beijing, made the following comments about Beijing's capacity to raise awareness about the HIV/AIDS threat: *"The Chinese government holds the power to ensure the cataclysm foretold by the UN never happens. A first step would be to unleash the full power of its propaganda apparatus, a huge machine that reaches the length and breadth of this vast country and penetrates into almost every pocket of society. Right now the machine is in high gear support of President Jiang's latest political theory, the Three Represents...On an even larger scale, enormous resources have been thrown into a campaign to smash the Falun Gong movement... Nothing like the same effort has been put into alerting people to the dangers of HIV/AIDS, say specialists in the field"* (FEER 15 August 2002)

HIV and AIDS

> *"The HIV/AIDS interventions are taking an extremely long time to implement due to the ignorance and highly conservative attitude of the government bodies* [in the PRC and TAR]. *Consider that the AIDS epidemic started 12 years ago (as a global epidemic) and the government* [still] *has no comprehensive intervention strategy. Hence Chinese and Tibetan people are extremely vulnerable."*
>
> – British aid worker who has experience in Tibet

A United Nations (UN) report published in June 2002, "HIV/AIDS: China's Titanic Peril" said that China is on the brink of an 'explosive' AIDS epidemic and could have 10 million infected people by the end of the decade.[19] The UN report cited *"insufficient political commitment"* and a *"scarcity of effective policies"* as undermining efforts to prevent the spread of the disease. The Chinese authorities state that in the first half of 2002, 1 million people in the People's Republic of China (PRC) had AIDS or were infected with the HIV virus, indicating that the authorities are becoming more aware of the scale of the epidemic.[20] Official recognition of the problem has been relatively recent in China, and linked to the fact that HIV is now affecting mainstream society – including the middle classes and the People's Liberation Army, as well as migrant workers and farmers in remote rural areas.[21]

While very few cases of HIV have been reported as yet in Lhasa, it has many of the preconditions for a 'very alarming' increase in the incidence of HIV in the near future.[22] Factors include low levels of awareness about HIV/AIDS, the influx of Chinese and other migrants from areas of China where an HIV epidemic is already emerging, and the rapidly expanding sex industry in Lhasa and other Tibetan urban areas. Low levels of education about the risks of AIDS make elements of the Chinese migrant and Tibetan community, including sex workers and their clients, particularly vulnerable. There is a clear link between the presence of an STI (sexually transmitted infection) and the transmission of HIV, for instance, and Lhasa has a high rate of STIs, including gonorrhoea and syphilis, although accurate statistics are not available.[23] Drug use is also an important factor in the transmission of AIDS, and poor hygiene practices as highlighted earlier in this report increase the risks.[24] Blood supply is another major problem, as blood in Tibet is not yet screened for HIV, although there are plans to initiate such screening in the TAR.

22 According to research undertaken by Tibet Public Health Bureau, Lhasa Public Health Bureau, Macfarlane Burnet Centre, August 2000

23 The Australia-based Macfarlane Burnet Centre has pointed to the high incidence of STIs in Tibet

24 The provinces of Xinjiang and Yunnan have the highest rates of HIV/AIDS in the PRC, primarily due to sharing of needles for drug use, although the virus is also spreading through sexual transmission

A western visitor to Shigatse in the TAR spoke to some sex workers in the city about their clientele and risks of AIDS.[25] The visitor reported to TIN:

> *"I met four young Tibetan women who had just arrived in Shigatse from a farming area near Lhasa just a few weeks before. All of them were illiterate. They said they have never had any STI, and if they did, they would have no idea how to get treatment. They said they never use condoms because they wash themselves after sex, but they did say they would use condoms if they were given to them. They didn't know anything about AIDS, though they had heard of it. Their charges were about 60 yuan (US$7.25), but for a whole night it is more, and the owner of the place where they worked keeps about half of this."*

A second Western source told TIN that they spoke to a group of Chinese sex workers who said the same as many of the Tibetan women, that you did not contract AIDS if you were hygienic. One of them said that they would only use a condom if their client 'looks sick'. The Chinese girls said their clients were Chinese, Tibetan, Nepali, Indian, and a small number of foreigners.

As in many other parts of the world, complex socio-economic and cultural factors have to be taken into account when assessing the policy framework for the containment of HIV and AIDS in Tibet. There is evidence that the authorities in Tibet are concerned about the threat of an HIV/AIDS epidemic, and are taking steps to develop preventive and educational strategies, some of which are being implemented with the help of western organisations.[26] In October 1999 a planning meeting was held in Lhasa attended by officials from Lhasa Municipality, and Lhokha and Shigatse prefectures to introduce participants to the issue of HIV and AIDS, and to discuss the development of a co-ordinated strategy on AIDS. At the meeting, the level of awareness regarding appropriate methods of control appeared to be very low; a video presentation included shots of police arresting prostitutes and a camp where people with HIV were isolated.[27] The film also depicted scenes of foreigners arriving in China or engaged in homosexual intercourse – a frequent tendency among Chinese officials has been to blame foreigners for the spread of HIV. The film apparently also gave an impression that simple improvements in hygiene, such as cleaning plates or disinfecting toilets, could be effective in controlling the spread of HIV and AIDS.

25 Full details of the conversations have been withheld in order to protect the identities of those concerned

26 The Chinese news agency Xinhua reported on 21 October 2002 that China has been engaged in 'co-operative efforts' with more than 30 international organisations, countries and regions in nearly 100 AIDS-related programmes. This co-operation had helped Chinese people *"to open their minds to new concepts"*, said Zhang Jianxin, a professor at Sichuan University, according to Xinhua. The professor said that attitudes towards AIDS are changing in China: *"Chinese people have come to realise that AIDS victims should not be blamed in terms of moral[ity]... It represents a breakthrough in AIDS education in China"*

27 This highlighted the concerns among health professionals in Tibetan areas that some highly vulnerable groups, such as drug-users and sex workers, can be singled out in a category of 'undesirables' by security personnel and may be subject to punishment such as detention in some instances rather than help and education

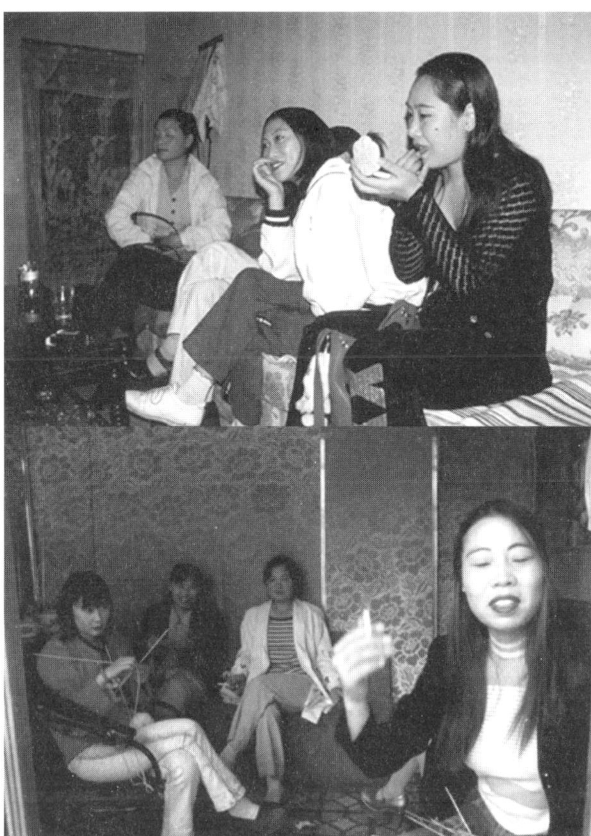

TOP a prostitute in a doorway, Lhasa © Barefoot Images
BOTTOM prostitute looking for business, Lhasa © Barefoot Images

Various meetings were held to follow up the October 1999 planning session, and in 2000 the first AIDS Awareness week was held in Lhasa. Free condoms were distributed to sex workers, and 'safe sex' messages, in both Chinese and Tibetan, were included in pamphlets and on graphic posters and banners. A further workshop was held in 2001, with representatives from Lhasa, Lhokha and Shigatse together with foreign health professionals, in order to draft a strategic plan to deal with HIV/AIDS in the region. According to Western health professionals working in the region, there is a commitment by the TAR authorities to raise community awareness about HIV, address blood and infection standards in clinical settings, and make condoms more available. Partially due to budgetary concerns and lack of capacity and expertise, however, there appears to have been little progress so far on implementation of the strategies under discussion.

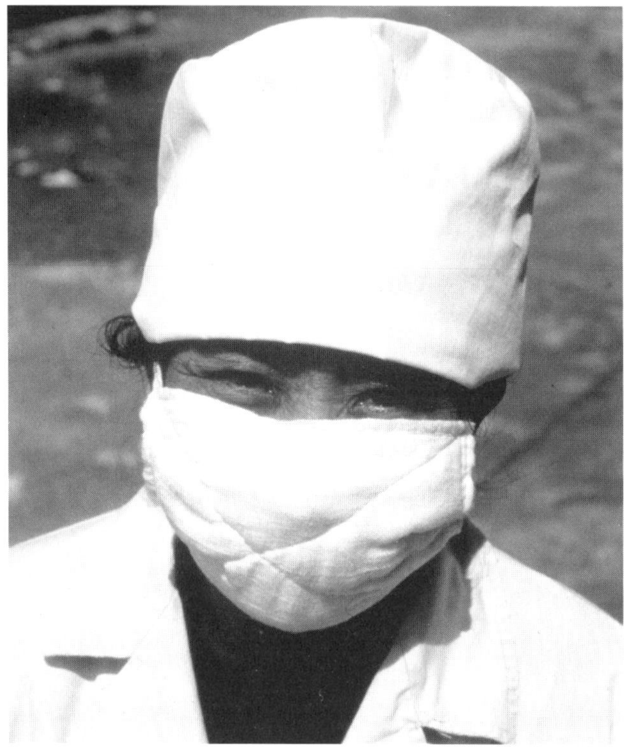

Tibetan doctor ©John Miles/Tibet Images

The Tibet Statistics Yearbook 2000 published by the TIbetan Statistical Bureau confirms that:

In 1999 – the year that the Western Development Scheme was announced – the number of hospitals in TAR dropped from 876 in 1998 to 824, hospital beds from 6305 in 1998 to 6255 in 1999, and the number of doctors from 5089 to 4696. These are gross numbers, not per capita figures.

Employment in the health care sector (called "Health Care, Sporting, and Social Welfare" in the Chinese statistics) was down from 14,200 in 1998 to 13,400 employees in 1999, which brings the total employees in this sector to a level much lower than that in 1990 (14,400). Given that Tibet has the most rapid population growth rate in China, this would amount to a sharp and significant reduction in per capita supply of infrastructure and personnel.

Conclusion

This report has shown that more than half a century after the incorporation of Tibet into the People's Republic of China (PRC), affordable and adequate health care is still not available to the majority of Tibetans. Many diseases that have been endemic to the Tibetan plateau for centuries are still not under control, emergency medical care is virtually non-existent, and the authorities are not yet taking decisive action in developing preventive strategies for newly emerging conditions such as HIV/AIDS.

During the 1990s, there was a reduction in Chinese state funding of health care as a proportion of total spending, while the costs of health care continued to increase, particularly in rural areas of Tibet and China. State spending on health tends to benefit a minority of people, who mostly live in urban areas of Tibet. This is consistent with the general pattern in China – according to one recent survey[1], 68% of Chinese government funding for health care goes towards looking after the wealthiest 20% of the population.

Beijing's economic development policy for the PRC's western regions, including Tibet, focuses on large-scale infrastructure projects such as roads, railways, dams and power stations. In comparison, 'soft' infrastructure projects – including health and education provision – are not prioritised in policy terms. Some Chinese economists have criticised this approach, suggesting that more attention should be paid to the development of human resources in western regions. Western medical professionals who have worked in Tibet confirm that the local authorities in Tibetan areas are tied into plans and targets set in Beijing, which do not take into account the unique circumstances in different parts of Tibet.

Tibet's health care system appears to be on a par with some of the poorest regions in developing countries, while in some eastern areas of China, health services that meet international standards have been provided for some years. The implementation of a health insurance system is a PRC policy that has been prioritised by President Jiang Zemin, in an attempt to address the crisis in rural health care throughout China. The Co-operative Medical System (CMS) in Tibet is providing some cover for Tibetans, but there are a number of issues to be addressed before it can be effective. The main reasons why Tibetans cannot receive adequate health care are related to education and training, standards of hygiene, affordability, accessibility and equality. While there are signs that the leadership in Beijing is acknowledging the national crisis in rural health care that developed following de-collectivisation and 'socialist modernisation' in the 1970s and 1980s, this report shows that there appears to have been little success in addressing the failures of health care provision in Tibet.

1 Harvard University health economist William Hsiao, quoted by Susan Lawrence in the Hong Kong-based publication "The Far Eastern Economic Review" 13 June 2002

Picture Captions

Front cover:

Trainee doctors learning to give injections, TAR
© Markus Bollen/Tibet Images

Back cover:

Box of dentist's tools
© Markus Bollen/Tibet Images

PLEASE NOTE:

In order to protect the identities of our sources, as well as their colleagues and friends in Tibet, it is not always possible or appropriate to reveal precise details of the location or subject matter that is being depicted in particular images

* the subject's identity has been obscured

CHAPTER ONE

page 10 montage:

(TOP LEFT) Shigatse hospital entrance

(TOP RIGHT) Shigatse Menze Khang (Tib. hospital)

(CENTRE) Queue at Tashilhunpo clinic, Shigatse

(BOTTOM) Basic medical centre near Mt Kailash
© Zonda/TIN

CHAPTER TWO

page 28 montage:

(TOP LEFT) Prices of drugs and medical treatment on display in a Tibetan hospital

(TOP RIGHT) Village dentist in eastern Tibet
© Markus Bollen/Tibet Images

(CENTRE RIGHT) Saying prayers for a sick man
© Jirina Simajchlova/Tibet Images

(BOTTOM) Tibetans in exile sorting traditional Tibetan medicine (TTM) pills in Dharamsala, India
© Diane Barker/Tibet Images

CHAPTER THREE

page 42 montage:

(TOP) Educational banner explaining toilet habits, on display in a medical centre in Shigatse
© Nick Dawson/Tibet Images

(CENTRE LEFT) Monastery supplies of yak butter
© Zonda/TIN

(CENTRE RIGHT) Unrefrigerated meat for sale in Shigatse market
© Zonda/TIN

(BOTTOM) An open-air Tibetan kitchen
© Zonda/TIN

CHAPTER FOUR

page 54 montage:

(TOP) Old man sleeping rough in Lhasa
© Barefoot Images

(CENTRE LEFT) Tibetan street child* outside TV shop
© Barefoot Images

(CENTRE RIGHT) Tibetan man scavenges for food from bin
© Barefoot Images

(BOTTOM) Beggar outstretched on a Lhasa street
© Barefoot Images

CHAPTER FIVE

page 66 montage:

(TOP LEFT) A new-born baby wrapped in a blanket at the Shigatse hospital in the TAR
© Catherine Platt/Tibet Images

(TOP RIGHT) Three babies sharing a hospital cot
© Irene Slegt/Tibet Images

(BOTTOM) Mother with son recovering from an operation at the Lhasa People's Hospital
© Catherine Platt/Tibet Images

CHAPTER SIX

page 74 montage:

(TOP) Tibetan with Kashin-Beck (Big Bone) Disease selling wild rhubarb
© Tim Nunn/Tibet Images

(BOTTOM LEFT) Abandoned syringes near a clinic

(BOTTOM RIGHT) Tibetan marmots – a factor in the spread of diseases such as the plague
© Zonda/TIN